Life, Love, and HIV

A Memoir

Jessica Ladeana Glaspie

ISBN: 978-0-578-85614-8

EBook ASIN: B08W6JGKBM

Author: Jessica Ladeana Glaspie

Illustrator: art_infinity

∽౿∼ **Special Thank You** ∽౿∼

I would first like to thank my three beautiful children for being my inspiration and pushing me to the finish line! Kaydence, Carter, and Jordan Patrick, you all are my entire world, and I am beyond blessed to be your Mom!

Secondly, I want to thank my Mom Rosita and my Stepdad Gerald, my Dad James Sr. and Stepmom Janice, for being the best support system a girl could ever ask for. You both have been my rock and always helped keep my head above water.

I want to thank my Sister Jennifer and my twin brother James Jr. for believing in me and staying by my side through all the ups and downs of my HIV journey.

Thank you to my Godparents Theresa and Joe! You both were there at the hospital with me and have been there ever since. I am forever grateful!

I want to thank my close friends that have been there to yell at me, laugh with me, and celebrate my successes. You all helped make this possible as well.

What was meant to break me made me unbreakable! I'm grateful for the lesson! So yes…let's get this show on the road!

Table Of Contents

✑ **Preface** ✑

I was the one that talked to the lonely kid in the corner that no one wanted to talk to and shared my food with people that I had no idea was hungry. I remember working with this guy at a call center in Georgia, and he used to join me for lunch all the time. I always used to get French fries because they were filling and cheap. Every time he sat with me, I'd offer him some. Most times, he declined, and I'd insist and say, "Go ahead! I won't eat 'em all!" After that phrase, he would actually eat them. It turned out he had a crush on me since we were in a training class, and it also turned out that…he was hungry.

Years later, he told me that I used to share my lunch with him when he had nothing to eat. I was so taken aback. I mean, it wasn't like I knew he was hungry. I was just polite. Plus, I hated eating in front of people, and they weren't eating too. I have always been that way. My parents raised me to be that way. They taught me that not everyone is fortunate, and not everyone can afford to eat a decent meal or have decent clothes and shoes that fit. I always went out my way to compliment someone because I learned that you never know what kind of day someone is having, and a simple "You look beautiful today," could actually be the reason they made it through one more day

I've always been a people person. I made Homecoming Court all four years of high school, and people used to be like, "How did she make it AGAIN?! For the third year in a row? She's ugly!" They were upset they didn't make the cut, and I did. Sometimes the grief that came with winning made it not even worth being on the ballot. I've come a long way. I've made it through tough times. It may not have been as tough as A LOT of other people, but it was still tough for me. Growing up, I'd never been without. It wasn't just me, though. I have a twin brother and older sister as well, so I guess the right thing to say is WE never went without. I don't recall having our lights cut off or no hot water or heat/Air Conditioning.

We never had to take public transportation outside of a school bus. My sister got a car at sixteen, so my brother and I barely took the bus the first couple of high school years. It's been an advantage and a disadvantage to not have to struggle. The disadvantage is that I don't know how to catch the city bus to this day, and I'm nervous to do so. I wouldn't know what to do if I had to go without heat or hot water. Hell, I don't even know how to change a flat tire! My point is, I don't know struggle like some people know the struggle, and I grind hard as hell to make sure my kids nor I ever have those experiences.

In the same sense, never having experienced those things always made me feel like I didn't have a story to tell…and then I contracted HIV. It has humbled me in more ways than anyone could ever imagine. It flipped this switch in my life, and I had to hit the ground running. I had to do something. And guess what? That person I talked to that was lonely in the corner, that person I shared my lunch with, that person I told was beautiful- have supported me in different ways from Q&As to Gala's to the AIDS Walk in Chicago. Some provided moral support when I needed it most. They have donated their time and their money in appreciation for me, just being me, doing things without expecting a reward.

What did Maya Angelou say? *"I've learned that people will forget what you said, people will forget what you did, but people will never forget how you made them feel."* God rest her soul because that phrase is a contribution to why I do the things I do. It's because of how I make people feel. When I make people feel good about themselves, it gives me purpose. It shows me that everything I went through and continue to go through today is not in vain. Thank you all for taking the time to read this book and follow my life as I go into depths that I've never gone into before…

This is my story...

This work depicts actual events in the life of the author as truthfully as recollection permits and/or can be verified by research. Occasionally, dialogue consistent with the character or nature of the person speaking has been supplemented. All persons within are actual individuals; there are no composite characters. The names of some individuals have been changed to respect their privacy.

Neither the author nor publisher will be held liable or responsible for any actual or perceived loss or damage to any person or entity, caused or alleged to have been caused.

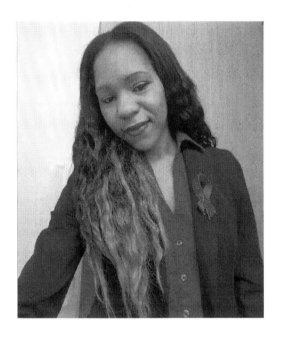

"In my life, there's been heartache and pain. I don't know if I can face it again. Can't stop now, I've traveled so far to change this lonely life. I wanna know what love is. I want you to show me. I wanna feel what love is. I know you can show me."

(Mariah Carey, I Want to Know What Love Is, Memoirs of an Imperfect Angel)

ᗡᕟ **The Quiet Storm** ᗡᕟ

I met him at a traffic light. I vividly remember what I had on that night and how inappropriate it was for it to be in the middle of January. It was this colorful, short sequins dress with these silver, peep-toe platform heels with a strap on the back. I had just dropped off a friend I met a few months earlier at her boyfriend's house and was on my way back home. *(We had gone to a club downtown Atlanta.)* It was 3:00–4:00 a.m., and I was sitting at the light waiting on my "Go" when this car pulled up to the right of me. At the time, I was driving my Godfather's Altima because I did not have a vehicle yet. His car was really nice. It was a Pewter colored 4 door Sedan with black rims and a loud sound system. I have always been into music, so anytime I got the opportunity to play it loud, I did. I naturally looked to my right when the car pulled up because I could see the headlights approaching.

Being aware of my surroundings was important in unfamiliar territory so I was always looking around me and in my mirrors. When you watch as much crime TV as I do, you become very aware of your environment. I turned back to watch for the green light, and when I looked to the right again, the driver had rolled his window down, signaling for me to do the same. I quickly snapped my head to the left as if I did not see him. I gripped the steering wheel tighter, watching the light, begging with my eyes for it to turn green. A part of me was terrified! I had watched one too many Lifetime movies that did not end so well.

My heart was beating fast, and my palms were sweating. I had only been in the Atlanta area for a little over six months, and I wanted to meet new people. I more so wanted to get over this guy I had just gotten out of a relationship with. I looked to my right again, and there he was, still motioning for me to roll my window down. All of this happened in a matter of seconds, but it felt like forever! My gut was telling me no. It was late, and I kept thinking, *"What the hell is he doing out at this time of the morning?"* Then, I said, *"Well, he's probably doing the same thing I'm doing! Leaving the club and heading home. Who knows?"* I went against my gut and rolled my window down. He said, *"What's ya name Shawty?"*

I told him the right name, although everything in me told me to say Jasmine. That was the fake name I used when I was not interested in someone that tried to holler at me. Then, he told me I was pretty and asked for my number. At this point, the light probably turned green, and yellow, and then red again. I kept looking over, and the light seemed like it never changed. He looked cute from a distance, and time was ticking. I then told myself to give him the wrong number, but being so pressed against time, I just chanced it and gave him the right number. And just like that, the light turned green, and we both went our separate ways.

He called me as soon as the highway divided us into two different directions and introduced himself as Darius. We talked the whole way home and every day after that for months. The first couple of months were great. What do they call it? The honeymoon phases? Yea, that's it. I started a journal, and it describes instances in my life from 2007 right up until today.

On March 11th, 2009, I briefly explained what this honeymoon phase was like. I wrote:

"Now I have a boyfriend. He's a Dope Boy (with a smiley face following.) Yes, he sells everything from drugs to TV's, but hey, he makes sure I'm straight, so it's whatever…He likes to go out and have fun, and he leaves everything up to me. Where we go, what we eat, everything. So far, we've been to the movies, dinner, and the park for a walk. Our first date was at 19th Street Café in Atlantic Station. He pulled out hundreds and fifties. I was like, 'Wow!' I stay weekends with him to get away from home. I love bein with him. Being at his house…"

Darius knew I loved pizza and orange pop, so he made sure he had it every time I was over. He bought me whatever I wanted whenever I wanted it. He made sure I got the, *"Good Morning Beautiful"* texts and the, *"Good Night"* phone calls. I was getting over a very serious relationship, which means that all of this probably wasn't as magnificent as I made it out to be, but nonetheless, I was living what I thought was the dream. It was the right place at the wrong time. Or maybe even the wrong place AND the wrong time.

There I was, twenty-one years old, intrigued by a lifestyle I had never experienced before.

I had never seen these drugs in real life. I had never seen a real handgun, **"tricks[1],"** and I had definitely never seen so much cash money in one place. The adrenaline rush that took over me when we were together was something I was thrilled to feel. I was addicted to it. I could not wait to get to him on the weekends and watch him sell to any and everybody. He did not live alone, though. He lived with two family members and his best friend. Imagine how much action was taking place there on a day-to-day basis. I could not wait to see them weighing little baggies and sorting pills. I was already sucked in, and we were only two months in.

I was not exposed to this kind of behavior growing up. My parents made sure of it. So, when I finally saw in front of my face what I had only seen in movies, I was enticed. I could not believe I missed out on all this excitement. My parents made sure my siblings and I had everything we wanted and needed. They were very particular about who we were allowed to be around and who could be around us. We grew up in a predominantly white, suburban area and attended predominantly white schools our entire lives. They wanted so much for us, and it was apparent. They worked hard to provide and made sure we knew the importance of working for what we wanted; and the importance of getting

---

[1] *A person who spends money on gratifying their sexual impulses and/or pleasures.* Urbandictionary.com

a higher education. That was all fine and good, but after being around Darius, I wanted to live the life he had exposed me to.

The life I knew was boring and unfulfilling. I wanted more, and he knew it. He groomed me so well. **I wrote:** *"He told me he wanted me to fall in love with him and that he's the last guy I'll ever be with. We'll see…"* The last guy I'll ever be with? That was extreme, but I was so vulnerable when I started messing with him that it probably wasn't far from the truth. He had the power to mold me into whoever he wanted me to be just to make him happy. I was trying to fill this void my ex had left, and I was looking for love in all the wrong places. I looked past so many red flags. A few months into our relationship, I learned three things: he had gone by two names, he lied about his age, and lied about what he did for a living. He told me his middle name the night we met, but never told me his first. He told me he was twenty-one when in fact, he was twenty, and he initially said to me that he worked for his sister's catering company.

I learned the truths really quick. Darius never came across as being aggressive or controlling when we were first together. He was so affectionate and so sweet. He was also very convincing, so I believed almost everything he told me. I thought he truly cared about me and that I was the only one. He just did not seem like the lying type, and I thought the world of him. Even after the truth came out, I downplayed the lies by saying, *"Well, at least he has money"* or *"Well, it's only a year he lied about."* My feelings grew strong in such a brief time. I wanted so badly to love someone else. I did not want to be a prisoner of love anymore, waiting on a relationship that was never going to be revived. I wanted to be committed and invested in someone else. I just wanted to move on.

The pain I experienced from losing that past relationship caused me to overlook so many things that I would not dare overlook today. We had rules in our relationship when it came to his "customers," especially the women. **"The trap**[2]**"** closed at Midnight when I was around. Point. Blank. Period. It worked for us. His phone went on silent, and there were no interruptions. Whether we wanted to have sex all night or just watch movies and chill, we could do that. Apparently, that's not how the drug game goes (I laugh about it now, but I was young back then.) One day I triggered him, and all hell broke loose. We were lying in bed, and his phone rang because he forgot to silence it. It was after Midnight, but he answered it anyway. Suddenly, he put his clothes on and made his way out the door to **"make a play**[3]**."** I was pissed! I put my clothes on also and went to my car to leave.

He came up to my car to ask me why I'm leaving. I stated, *"You said the trap closed at Midnight! It's 2 in the morning!"* And he just spazzed. He started yelling and cursing, telling me that he has to make money and I need to "fall back," etc. He was screaming in my face, so I pushed

---

[2] *A place where drugs are sold. Urbandictionary.com*
[3] *Sell something to someone.*

him back, then he shoved me. I hit him after that because I felt the need to defend myself, and then BOOM! He slammed me on the hood of my car. That was the first time a man had ever put their hands on me, and I did not know how to take it. So, I called 911. I ended up leaving before the police got there. On my drive home, I just cried and cried. Was it worth all of this? All I kept thinking was that my ex would NEVER do that to me.

The person I saw Darius become that night was someone I never wanted to see again. I was dealing with so much grief, I could not contain my anger and frustrations any longer. As much as I seemed happy, I wasn't. I wanted my relationship back with my ex. I told myself I was never talking to Darius again. I was quiet with him because I was observant. I was an analyst by nature, always observing and analyzing people and my environments, and acting accordingly. Plus, I really needed to feel him out because I did not want to get my heart broken again. He was dealing with many things I had not learned about until later in our relationship. He internalized everything until you took him there. I was also dealing with a lot of things and internalizing them.

Together, we were the perfect storm…like a hurricane, silently building its momentum before making landfall. The disaster was about to strike, and I had NO clue what I was getting myself into. All I knew was what I wanted to get myself out of…, and that was this relationship. How did I get here? It all started in 2005 when I met my ex in college.

The end of that relationship was the beginning of my worst nightmare…

"And maybe I can take you out (sometimes) so let's exchange digits and later arrange visits, either your place or mine, yea. This a different type of commitment, I'm talkin bout a true friendship, someone I can depend on to be down no matter what…"

(Musiq, B.U.D.D.Y, Luvanmusiq)

∽ **First Comes Love** ∽

I met the ex I spoke of in 2005 while moving into my college dorm. It was literally the first day of my freshman year. I was walking down the hall in these navy-blue short shorts with socks that came right up to the middle of my calves, and a white tank top. I knew I was cute, and no one could tell me any different. The dorm I chose was co-ed and had all levels of undergraduate students. I mean, I wasn't going to select the all-freshman dorm because I wanted access to everybody, especially the ones that had already been there and knew where to go and where all the hot spots were. This was my first taste of real freedom. This was my first time being on my own, away from my parents and siblings. This was my first time having the ability to do whatever I wanted at whatever time I wanted to do it.

From birth until this very day, I had someone telling me what I can and cannot do and who I can and cannot see. All I thought was, *"Today, all of that goes out the window!"* The adrenaline that soared through my body was like skydiving from an airplane, anxiously waiting to release my parachute. I was so nervous about being on my own, yet so excited to finally get this taste of independence I had been waiting my whole life to have. Our suite was at the end of the hall, and every other suite was of the opposite sex. Next to us were boys, and the suite next to that were girls (and so on and so forth.) I was rooming with a friend from high school (who remains one of my best friends today). A few suites down was a boy that caught my eye as soon as I walked by him. He was light-skinned with braids and a smile that could just light up the world. I saw him from a distance and was sure to walk slow when passing him in the hallway.

I wanted him to notice me without being conspicuous, so I walked very casually back and forth a few times. The residence hall was chaotic, to say the least. Parents were moving their kids in, and a team of volunteers helping with move-in day was cascading through the hallways. Movers and Shakers are what they were called. There were incentives for volunteering, so there were way more movers than necessary. The suites were made so that only four people shared one bathroom versus a community-style living where the entire hall (and sometimes the whole floor) shared the one. That was one thing I was sure I did not want when looking for colleges to attend. I was NOT going to share a bathroom with an entire floor of people.

Anyways, I spoke to him on the way to my room and counted the suites between us to know what door to knock on later in the day. (Yes, I already had my eye on the prize. Plus, I was ready to party!) There were only two suites in-between us; it was perfect! After my roomy and I got settled in and our parents finally left, we were ready to start living the, "college life." We walked to their suite and introduced ourselves. My roommate was shy, but I was so outspoken.

I managed to get his name and learned he was from the area and knew where all the hotspots were. His name was Alex. I don't remember the first time I slept with him, but I know for sure that he was my "Cutty buddy" by the end of the semester. In other words, the person I called in the middle of the night for one thing and one thing only, sex.

Do not act like you have never had someone you called for a fix! His sex was like a drug; so good, so addicting. I never had intentions of being in an actual relationship with him, considering how we started. We understood the roles we played and were okay with where we stood. On drunk nights, after the parties or the club, I called Alex. Up late doing homework and studying, I called Alex, took a "break," and then went back to studying. He was my go-to, and I was his. Hell, we were freshmen in college living the dream with no rules, nobody to tell us to go to bed or get up, and nobody to stop us from making ALL the terrible decisions we were bound to make.

Nobody in their right mind wanted to be in a committed relationship at that time in their lives; Not people like myself anyway who grew up with way more restrictions than necessary. No one told us not to EVER take an 8:00 a.m. class when you are a freshman, so you can only imagine how many absences we had for those courses. Alex and I both had an 8:00 a.m. class that we missed numerous times because we were up all-night partying and having sex. This went on the first and second semester and throughout the summer. By sophomore year, I started to get emotionally attached, but he no longer attended the university. His roommate was still there, so I continued to see a lot of Alex.

By this time, my roommate, my suitemates, and I moved into the on-campus apartments, which were larger and more fun. Alex was always at the parties with his friend and almost always returned to my apartment afterward. I shared a room for just a little while, but one of my roommates got pregnant and moved back home, allowing the rest of us to have our own rooms. It was strange how connected Alex and I were because I had never felt that connection with any other person. The chemistry we had was insane, and the conversations were always endless. We would be up until the wee hours of the morning texting or talking or just hanging out. By the end of sophomore year, I wanted to pursue a relationship.

We spoke on the phone late nights and early mornings for quite some time, and he spent a lot of time with me on and off-campus. I felt like if we were already mutually exclusive, why not have the title too? He had an ex that went to a sister school of ours not too far away, and I could tell she was the reason he was hesitant about getting in a relationship. She was his high school sweetheart, and I cannot say that he had officially let that go by this time. Regardless, I wanted him, and I wanted him all to myself. I was nineteen when we FINALLY decided to become a couple and was SUPER EXCITED to change my relationship status on my social media to "In A

Relationship." It was July 18th, 2007, to be exact. The decision came about subtly via text messages.

I wrote about it in my journal, and the entry went like this:

"I have the most EXCITING news… My relationship status on my social media says, 'In a Relationship' YIKES! It really happened. We're finally together, and I am soooooooo happy…Let me tell you how it happened; We were texting each other like we always do, and he asked a sarcastic question and said, 'You really wanna date me?' I was kind of irritated because he was taking it for a joke, and I was serious. That's what I told him, and he said, 'Let's do it,' and I got the biggest smile on my face and replied, 'Let's…"

It sounds pretty lame, I know, but I wanted this so bad. In my freshman year of college (2005), I decided to make scrapbooks. I had pictures and fliers from every party we went to and random nights in our dorms. I wanted to journal, though, so I could remember how I felt throughout my college journey. In 2007, I decided to start keeping a journal. Here I am, fourteen years later, and I still write. I do not write every day as I did back then, but often. It has been one of the better decisions I have made over the years as it allows me to go back and really feel today how I felt back then. Anyhow, it was like I won the lottery when I got with Alex.

I was home for the summer, about five hours away from him, when we finally decided to be together. I could not

WAIT to get back to school. I was thinking about all the memories we would make and the fun we would have once I moved back on campus. I thought about movie nights and dinner dates. I thought about all the college parties we would now attend as a "couple" and all the girls and boys that would be staring at us with envy. I couldn't contain the excitement, and August couldn't come fast enough.

Well, August came and went, as did the rest of the school year. Our relationship was…. juvenile. We argued over the stupidest things. I was super jealous and needy for attention, and he was super calm, laid-back, and did not care for the attention. That definitely did not work in my favor. I was the type to be mad when he did not answer his phone nor call back. I would immediately send text messages like, *"Where are you that you can't answer your phone?"* or, *"I've called you twice? What are you doing?"* I'll admit, I was defensive and annoying, and I did not realize it until years later. I wanted the relationship so bad that I was afraid of losing it when I finally got it.

I learned that a lot of guys do not like insecure women. I mean, if you are not confident in yourself, how are you confident in your relationship? But when you are a nineteen-year-old college student, who the hell cares about that. I was as insecure as they came. I was still skinny with no hips, no ass, and no boobs. In my mind, lacking those three things meant I had to be super overprotective and overbearing when it came to my boyfriend. Like, do not even GLANCE at another woman! It was silly, but it was real. I always felt like the next girl was prettier than me, and for that reason, I was easily attached and overzealous. Since Alex was no longer a student, he lived in a city about thirty-five minutes away with his parents.

He stayed a lot of nights at the apartment, though. So much that he ended up moving in with my roommates and I. They did not mind him being there, and I definitely did not mind going to bed with him every night and waking up to him every morning. I did mention that our relationship was juvenile, right? I'm sure most relationships were at that age. I wrote about so many instances in our relationship where I went off on him about something so petty and stupid.

One week into our relationship, I wrote:

"Some girl put a comment on Alex's social media talkin about this girl wasn't lying when she told her how sexy he is. I was like, excuse me? That's soooooo rude! She sees that he's clearly in a relationship, and she gon flirt like that on public internet. Fuck dat. I ain't goin…"

Two weeks into the relationship, it was:

"Alex was supposed to call me after he got done smokin. He didn't. This was around Midnight. Well, by like 1:45 a.m., he hadn't called back, so I called, and he ain't answer. I was instantly pissed. AND he didn't call back. I texted him and said I would love to know why it was takin him 2 hours to smoke AND why he didn't answer his phone. No text back…"

What in the entire hell?!!! Who acts like that? I laugh now, but that was very toxic. I was way too insecure, and I **projected**[4] all my insecurities onto him. I just liked him so much, and I didn't want to allow anyone to slide in and snatch him from me. We had many conversations like the one I wrote about, and I made a lot of noise about things I should have been quiet about. Talk about growth! I would not make an issue about those things today, but it took me years to gain the confidence necessary to have a healthy relationship.

We did have a ton of good nights and good memories, though. He made my college experience memorable. The sex was bomb, he was a lot of fun to be around, and I absolutely loved his entire family. I met his family before we were officially together when I was visiting for the 4th of July in 2007. His parents were high school sweethearts and perfect role models for us. He had two brothers, both younger than him, and they were such a ball of joy. There was an artist that came out the year we started dating named Soulja Boy. One thing about living in the St. Louis metro area was that they could DANCE. They knew how to do all the current dances, and the "Superman" dance was one of the most popular.

The first time I saw it, I was at Alex's house, and his little brothers showed me how to do it to the song. I loved being over there. His family was always so inviting and friendly.

---

[4] A *type of defense mechanism that people use by unintentionally externalizing difficult emotions and putting them onto others (footnote?).*

I still think about them whenever that song comes on. By December, we were saying, *"I Love You's"* and fuckin like jackrabbits. I noted several times that we should be using condoms before something bad happens but rarely did condoms come into play. I never wanted us to end, and no one could tell me that we would ever be over. I mean, first comes love, then comes marriage, right?

"People see it now asking all about me, and how they always thought we were so perfect together. Let's re-write the end, start over again, and it's gon go better now. Cause when Im looking in your eyes, feels like the first time. Give me one good reason why, we can't just press rewind"

(Mariah Carey, For the Record, E=MC2)

～ **Then Comes A Baby Carriage?** ～

I won't elaborate on how amazing our sex life was but just know, it was pretty fucking amazing. Alex and I would do it anytime, anywhere, and several times a day. It was good every. single. time.

On December 16th, 2007, I wrote:

"We kicked it at Tyler's crib on Thursday night. Got drunk and shit. Came back and had sex...He was layin on his back in my bed, and I just went for it...I think we were both lost in the heat of the moment cuz we were doin some freaky shit..."But you know what happens when you get too comfortable, right? With the absence of condoms AND birth control, we were risking it all by engaging in unprotected sex with the pull-out method nowhere to be found.

I continued to say:

"I'm always afraid that I'm gonna get pregnant. But if I did, I wouldn't care. I'd be happy. I want to have his kids one day... life just seems to be so much easier once you're pregnant. You get more money from the government. I can go home and get low-income housing or Section-8 and live basically rent-free. And Alex can come with me...I know I wanna get pregnant and drop out of school and live a normal life..."

When I say I look back at these journal entries and shake my head! My idea of normal back then was misconstrued. I learned that when you hang around certain people all the time, you normalize certain behaviors that you continuously see. A lot of my friends at the time were pregnant or had babies already. I felt like I was missing out on so much having to go to school. I was upset with my parents for quite some time for making me go to college when at the time, they hadn't gone themselves. My friends with kids (or pregnant) had their own place for next to nothing and received food stamps. I was in college, struggling to make my meal plan last, and living with roommates. I wanted out, and I thought getting pregnant was the only way. With that being said,

by January 11th, 2008, I was pregnant. I wrote:

"I'm pregnant. Yes, my love, I said it. I'm about five weeks due September 16th. Can you believe it? You probably can after everything I have told you...lol. I found out Wednesday morning. I took a home pregnancy test, and it was positive. Then yesterday I went to the doctor to be sure and sure enough, positive again..."

I remember feeling scared but excited at the same time. I remember thinking how pissed off my parents were going to be because I was only twenty and wasn't even close to being done with college. Alex was scared about what his parents were going to say too. But after he told them, and they didn't flip, he was excited. He said, *"Sweetheart, we're about to have a baby,"* and my stomach dropped. The reality of having a baby was terrifying. I had NO clue how to be a mother, and I wasn't around my friends long enough to learn any parenting skills. I know my parents were more disappointed in me because they wanted me to focus on school, and there I was about to have a baby.

I remember telling my mom that Alex was going to join the Air Force and that we would get married. I remember telling her I would finish school after I had the baby. She didn't really hear none of that, but it happened, and there was nothing anyone could do to change it. My mom called back and told me I needed to get an abortion and finish school. However, that was not an option for me. I was against the whole idea of abortions. Especially since the sex was consensual and I was in a committed, **monogamous relationship**[5]. I kept telling her there was no way I was doing that.

I know she was just scared for me and wanted me to finish getting my bachelor's degree, but I just couldn't bring myself to abort a baby. However, God had different plans for us. Exactly one week after finding out I was pregnant, I miscarried our baby. Can you imagine what that journal entry was like? I wrote about it in great detail.

On January 24th, 2008, at 9 p.m., I wrote:

"I have so much to tell you. I got a baby book and prenatal pills and a parenting magazine from my Gyno, Dr. Smith. I was so excited...We talked about how spoiled our baby was

---

[5] *Having only one spouse, one sexual partner, or one mate.* Dictionary.com

gonna be, and Alex kept sayin 'He' so clearly, he wanted a boy. This went on for a week, and then BAM...I had a miscarriage one week after I found out I was pregnant. I started bleeding, and I thought my period came because I was having stomach and back pains too. So, I called my mom, but she was in Bible Study. So, I called Alex's mom, and she's like, 'Well technically, you're not supposed to have any bleeding while you're pregnant,' and I just started tearing up.

I couldn't get a hold of Alex to go to the hospital cuz he was in the gym. So, I waited like an hour for him to come home, and we went to the emergency room around 9 p.m. I waited like 20 minutes after filling out paperwork, and before I knew it, I was naked under a hospital gown, and nurses were drawing blood. I threw up after that. I just got nauseous. I was in excruciating pain in my lower abdomen and back. I couldn't sit still for nothing. After I vomited, I went to sleep, waiting on test results. I prepared for the worst but hoped for the best, and sure enough, I lost my baby..."

Anyone who has experienced a miscarriage or loss of a child can understand the devastation I felt when this happened to me. I was so in love, and I just knew this was meant for us. I couldn't believe God did not allow this to happen for me. At the end of that entry, I wrote that I loved him, and I hope he still wanted to marry me even though I lost our baby. Read that again. I blamed myself for that miscarriage. I was guilt-tripping so hard, I felt inadequate.

I felt like I had let Alex down and did not know how to psychologically process what I was experiencing. If I could go back, I would seek counseling and talk to someone about it. The process of miscarrying a child can be so damaging physically and emotionally. I was probably more emotionally challenged than anything else. Still, there was such a huge stigma back then about seeing a psychotherapist that I didn't want to see one. I did not want anyone to judge me, and I did not want my friends and family to think I was overreacting.

I honestly did not know I was grieving. I wasn't sure exactly what was going on. I just know I wanted space from Alex. I didn't want him around so much. I did not want to be bothered by people, and I remember skipping all my classes over the next few days. I honestly feel like that is when our relationship started going downhill. *I became very anti-social and withdrawn, and I cried during random times of the night. I couldn't sleep well, and I wasn't eating right. These were very common symptoms of* **Major/Clinical Depression,** but I had no idea.

It would be years before I was diagnosed. Over the next few days, my mom pressured me to get on Birth Control. I lied and told her I was scheduled to start birth control, so she would leave me alone, but the truth was that I wasn't. I didn't want to get on birth control, and now that I lost a pregnancy, I wanted another one. I know it sounds absolutely insane, but once you wrap your mind around something like that, it's hard to get it out of your head. I kept writing about what our life would be like with a baby and how we would get married. I was only twenty years old. Now that I look back on all of this, I think I just felt like having a baby with him would ensure he could never leave me.

I was so narrow-minded. Here I am today with three kids and a single mom. I had it all wrong back then, but you couldn't tell me that. On February 18th, 2008, I took another pregnancy test because my period had never come from the last miscarriage. My mom kept asking me if my cycle came because she knew I couldn't start birth control until after my first period after the miscarriage. I kept telling her no, and she immediately assumed I was pregnant again. Alex and I didn't stop having unprotected sex after the first miscarriage.

We probably should've, but I didn't care if I got pregnant again. I was wrapped up in the idea of being a mom. Anyway, my test came back positive again.

On February 21st, I wrote:

*"On Monday, I took 2 tests. The first one I took early in the morning and that test was positive. Then, I drank a whole bunch of fluids, and the 2nd one was negative. So, I went to the doctor yesterday, and they said the pee test was slightly positive. Either I'm really early in my pregnancy, or there's still residual from the miscarriage. So, they drew my blood to check my **HCG level**[6], and there you have it..."*

---

[6] *Your pregnancy hormone*

This time, we tried to keep the pregnancy to ourselves. I had to tell my mom because she was already on my ass about getting on birth control. She was disappointed all over again, but I still wasn't getting an abortion. This time more people were FOR an abortion than against one.

The first miscarriage had already taken a destructive toll on our relationship, so I couldn't imagine what this pregnancy would do. It was either going to make us or break us. It was St. Patrick's Day, and I went for my first ultrasound. They had set my due date for November 10th. On March 26th, I went for a second ultrasound. At the first one, they didn't detect a heartbeat and couldn't tell if it was too early. This time, the baby hadn't developed any more than the weeks before, and there was no heartbeat still. The doctor told me that I was going to miscarry again. They gave me an option to wait a week to see if I would miscarry naturally or to provide me with a **D&C**[7] and have them remove what had developed.

I chose the D&C. I had the surgery on March 27th, and by April 3rd, I was a single woman. Let me just say I was raging with emotions, and I didn't know how to handle everything I was going through. I had broken up with Alex over messages I found between him and his ex on social media. It was foolish and one of my biggest regrets when I realized what I did and tried to make amends. I was angry because I was going through miscarriages, and he was

---

[7] *Dilation and Curettage. A surgical procedure performed by scraping the uterine wall*

entertaining this girl. I was still trying to process everything that was happening, and I was going about it the best way I could. There is no right or wrong way to grieve, but society can sometimes change that dynamic if you allow it.

I became very insecure in the relationship after losing our babies. (As if I wasn't insecure enough already.) He left his social media page logged in, and I couldn't help but read all the messages. I was feeling very insignificant by this time. I thought I couldn't have kids, and that would for sure be a turn-off for him. I felt like he had every reason in the world to start looking elsewhere. The truth was, he had no interest in being with anyone else at that time. My self-doubt was the reason I walked away from the relationship and the reason he refused to take me back.

Yes, I said take me back because I fought to have that relationship back for YEARS. It's said that anything worth having is worth fighting for, and I fought like hell. In June 2008, I decided to move to Atlanta. I know, I know. Random as hell! It was supposed to be for the summer. I needed a break from that life. I had just had two miscarriages and lost the one person I just knew would be mine forever. I thought that me going to Georgia for the summer would be good for us. I thought it would allow us to miss each other and start fresh when summer was over. I have never been so wrong. You know the saying, "Out of sight, out of mind?"

That's how it felt when I left Illinois for Atlanta. When I left, he had written me a letter, and in the letter, he promised me he would be there when I got back. He said he's not going anywhere and that he didn't have a ring yet but that it was coming in the near future. I held on to those promises for so long. Thinking back on it now, it was so much false hope. I was convinced we would make it work by the time I went back to Illinois, but Alex had different plans. He was cautious with me. He would get me to the edge, but he was careful not to push me. By that, I mean I was always within his reach. When he wanted me, I was there. I believed everything he told me. Every promise he made I held near and dear to my heart. To me, he could do or say no wrong.

Our communication was so off after being in Atlanta for just a few weeks. He would text or call me every day when I first got there, but those messages and calls were few and far between after a few weeks. I would tell him I want space and leave me alone for a little while and then get upset when he actually did it. Poor Alex. I was an emotional wreck. The miscarriages messed me up. He didn't know how to handle me, and truthfully, I could barely handle myself. My journal entries are prime examples of just how unsure of myself I really was. On July 9th, 2008, I wrote about how I expressed to him that I wasn't feeling this whole non-communication thing, and he's like, *"You wanted 'space,' and I'm giving it to you, and now that's not what you want. Jessica, what do you want me to do?"*

I spent the rest of the summer regretting ever telling him I wanted space, time to myself, to be left alone, etc... I didn't mean it. I thought my absence would make him miss me more, call me more…Nope. Distance makes the heart grow fonder; they say. That didn't exactly work in my favor either. I ended up not going back to Illinois to finish school. By August, Alex and I were done, so I had no desire to go back to Illinois ever again. I wanted to transfer and finish college in Georgia. I "broke" the news to him, thinking he would be hurt that I was never coming back, but his silence spoke volumes. I started working two jobs to keep my mind off everything that was going on in my life. I worked in a call center full time and a retail store part-time. I worked A LOT. Monday thru Friday at my full-time job and nights, weekends, and holidays at the retail store.

I struggled with having idle time and an idle mind because I would overthink EVERYTHING. I worried myself to death about EVERYTHING. I was falling prey to another mental illness, and again, I had no idea. **Anxiety disorder**[8] was starting to take over, and I didn't write for months. I was devastated my relationship was over. I wanted so badly for it to work. I had never felt so lost. When I finally wrote in December of the same year, I found out that Alex was talking to someone else and got in a relationship with her when I left. It all made sense. How could he continuously communicate with me when he was interested in someone else? All I remember thinking was, *"Man, I really fucked this one up."*

---

[8] *Anxiety disorders differ from normal feelings of nervousness or anxiousness, and involve excessive fear or anxiety.* psychiatry.org

I went through her social media. I tried to make it all make sense, like, *"Maybe she's this? Or maybe she's that?"* You know how you instantly start to compare yourself to someone else when you're not over someone? I was driving myself CRAZY. She was very pretty and seemed to be well put together. I was desperate to know what she had that I didn't. Yes, desperate. At this point, there was no love, no marriage, and no baby in a baby carriage. I was so down about it. I needed a pick-me-up, and I needed it BAD.

"Over and over again, you fell in love with your best friend. Shoulder to shoulder with him, Bonnie and Clyde to the end. right here, right now. You should tell him how he changed your life, right here, right now. You should tell him thank you every night. Right here, right now, grab that man and hold him tight. Right here, right now. You will love him till the day you die"

(Lyfe Jennings, Right Now, Tree of Lyfe)

∞ **Like A Ton Of Bricks** ∞

The news of my ex moving on at the end of 2008 had me praying for a better 2009. I wanted to start over. I wanted to start finding myself again and letting go of what was. I looked forward to the New Year! I brought in the New Year at a popular Atlanta nightclub with a guy friend I had met a few weeks earlier. We had a ball. We drank and laughed and danced all night long. There was a champagne toast and balloon drop at Midnight, and it was the first time I had ever experienced that. For the first time in a long time, I was having fun, and I was as carefree as I could be. After that night, I just knew my year was going to be amazing! Rumor had it that how you bring in the new year is how your year will go. That was a pretty good sign for me!

Two days later, everything changed, and devastation came knocking AGAIN. We were very, very close to our Grandparents on my Dad's side. They were from Mississippi. They were so loving, and understanding and they loved us through the good, the bad, and the ugly like most Grandparents do. They were the glue to our family. Every Christmas Eve, we spent the evening there laughing, eating, and making good memories. It was the one time of the year that we all came together. Aunties, uncles, cousins, children, and grandchildren were able to put all of our problems aside and have a good time. Christmas Eve of 2008, I missed "Christmas at Grandma's."

I was so far away and did not plan to go back home after moving just six months earlier. It would end up being the last Christmas I spent with my grandfather, my PaPa. On Saturday January 3rd, my sister called to tell me that my PaPa wasn't doing well. The doctors stated he might not make it through the day. She was crying hysterically and barely breathing. I was stuck in Atlanta trying to find same-day flights so that I could say a final goodbye. It's always cold and snowing in Chicago at this time of year, so my flight got delayed. I arrived around 10:30 that night, and my PaPa was lying in the hospital bed in so much pain.

It's the last thing I remember about him. I remember not knowing what to say to him and being afraid to touch him. He was frail and was moaning and grunting in excruciating pain. I wanted so bad to take the pain away, but I couldn't. He had been suffering for quite some time, and I know he didn't want to suffer anymore. He made it through the night even though the doctors thought he wouldn't. He was one of the strongest men I had ever known.

I stayed a couple of days and visited more. I flew back to Atlanta that Monday to be ready for work on Tuesday. The Operations Manager grabbed me off a call around 9:30 a.m. My Dad asked my job to inform me that my PaPa had passed away. I felt my knees go weak as I broke down crying. I thought, *"I was JUST there! I should have stayed just one more day."* I felt guilty for being so far away. I felt even more guilty for leaving him there and going back to Atlanta. I didn't want PaPa to die alone. My biggest fear to this day is dying alone. January 6th of that year, he was gone. I was sick about it. Imagine having to deal with death amid a storm that already felt unbearable? I was at my wit's end, and I wasn't sure how much more I could take.

I wasn't handling PaPa's death well and was still grieving over a love I couldn't accept was lost. All these holes being punched in my heart, and nothing or no one seemed to fill them. I couldn't drink them away. I couldn't smoke them away. All I could do was write them away, so I continued with my journal entries, which (unsurprisingly) saved my sanity. Writing has always been therapy for me, whether it was poetry or writing in my journal. Right before PaPa passed, I started conversing with a guy named Desmond. It all started from a comment he put on one of my pictures from the New Year's party I mentioned earlier. It was short and sweet, *"Over there slapped Lol."*

It was a picture of me in this little black dress that fit all the tiny curves I had. I was holding a drink in my hand, stirring it, and cracking up about who knows what. I responded with a quick, *"You already know...lol,"* and the conversation went on from there. We somehow managed to start messaging each other privately and ended up exchanging numbers. I had met him a couple of years prior through a friend of mine from college. We didn't talk much, so I barely knew him, but we were friends on the internet, and you can learn A LOT about someone from their social media. Anyway, we hit it off pretty hard and moved pretty fast.

We tried for a relationship back then, but me being on such an emotional rollercoaster never allowed for a relationship to prosper. I was hurting so bad, and all I wanted was comfort in the midst of all this pain. Desmond gave that to me at a time when I needed it the most. I wrote about him several times and detailed our sexual encounters. The first encounter was at a beach resort the night of my PaPa's funeral. The funeral was that morning, and Desmond made sure that I was okay from the day he died. He was the only one I wanted to talk to.

We had been conversing since New Year's, and he ended up taking the train to stay with me that night. We were both pretty nervous about meeting because we hadn't seen each other in a while. It was freezing and snowing, so I know he thought it had better be worth the trip! And me? Well, I was thinking the same thing! I think it's safe to say that it was worth all the hours, minutes, seconds, and gas! We started with a few drinks to knock the edge off and maybe calm our nerves. We both brought our laptops for music, and before I knew it, our clothes were off, and the foreplay was just getting started. He was good at EVERYTHING.

His oral sex was beyond belief, and the sex almost had me packing my shit and moving in with him. I was comfortable with him, and he made me feel like I had known him forever. He was gentle and treated me like precious cargo. He touched softly and kissed tenderly. I couldn't help but be so vulnerable with him. I don't know how long we tangled in the bedsheets, but it was morning before I knew it. We got up and went to church the next day, and I remember us laughing so hard about it making jokes about having to repent for the night before. I guess a little dark humor, but whatever it took to keep my mind off PaPa, I was all for it.

After church, we went back to my mom's house for dinner and just chilled until it was time for him to catch his train back home. We were sitting on two different couches across from each other, sending texts that said, *"I miss you already, and you're not even gone."*

On March 11th, I wrote:

"He was about to have me on some stupid shit. Droppin out of school, moving back to Illinois so we could be together. He has a job making (however much) an hour, and he was saying he wanted me to move back so he could take care of me..." Desmond was always there when it counted. He was the only person outside of my family that consoled me after my PaPa's death. I called Alex crying. He talked to me briefly, but I could tell he wasn't good at being supportive about it and was having a hard time supporting the conversation. I called my close friend Sydney and left a voicemail on her phone crying and crying. I damn near begged for a callback, but I never got one until the day before his funeral.

I was very angry about that for such a long time. I was there for so many people, but where were they now that I needed them the most? I was a thousand miles from those that cared most and dealing with these incidents alone took a toll on me. I knew I had my Godparents, and I knew I had

Desmond. I always had him, and to this day, he is still in my corner. I often think about what could have happened between us had I been in a better space mentally and emotionally. I guess the world may never know!

April Fool's Day had rolled around, and I used it as an opportunity to reach out to my ex. I was always looking for a reason to contact him. I found myself always trying to figure out if he still thought about me, still loved me, or even just missed me a little. I texted him how much I missed him and how much I still loved him. I had every intention of telling him, *"April Fools!"* even though it was 100 percent the truth. He texted me back that he missed me too, and so I said, *"Aprils Fools lol,"* and he tried to play it off the same way I did. It was so corny! I couldn't believe I even did it. But the conversation kept going, and before I knew it, I was on my way to Memphis to see him play in a baseball tournament. I drove six hours to see this man for ONE night.

I was absolutely looney for that! I went to such great lengths to try to win him back; it was borderline obsessive and, not to mention, pathetic. I'm glad I can laugh about it now but back then, it hurt so bad to still be in love with someone that may never love you the same. That was the last time I had seen him until about Halloween of that year when he told me he was having a baby. DEVASTATION AGAIN!!!! I was in Illinois that weekend for fun and had hit him up just to talk. We got on the subject of his relationship, and I asked him what she knew about me. Apparently, she didn't know much, but she knew that I had miscarried twice and that we used to live together. So, I asked if he had ever gotten her pregnant.

I have no clue why I even wanted to know that, but I did. He just looked at me. He didn't answer, so I asked again, and yet again, he looked at me and put his head down. At this point, I assumed it was a yes, so I just asked what happened. He continued to look down, and so I said, *"Is she pregnant right now?!"* And he kept his head down and said, *"Yeah."* I could not believe it. I lost it.

On November 2nd, 2009, I wrote:

"He kept askin if I was good, and I'm like yeah. But he knew I wasn't. So, he kept askin, and I finally broke down after he got out the car. (I was in the driver seat, ready to pull off) and he said, 'Can I at least get a hug?' I hugged him and cried like a baby. Hurt that we weren't able to have ours, but she gets to keep hers. Hurt that everybody knows but me...I felt so stupid. So, I emailed him and told him how I felt and said I wasn't calling anymore, but he can call if he wants to talk. I told him I didn't hate him and that I wasn't mad (which was the polite thing to do...) I texted him and told him to check his email, and he responded and said 'okay,' and the signature on his text was <6/23/2010>. That must be her due date. He seems so excited, you know?"

I don't know why I expected anything less than excited when she got pregnant. Alex was always good with kids (he was a great big brother,) and his Dad was a great role model for his boys. For so long, I tried to understand why I lost my pregnancies and why I couldn't be the first to have his child.

When I got pregnant, I had hoped for a girl because Alex has all brothers. So, when I lost both pregnancies, I was disappointed in more ways than one. However, now I see why things happened the way that they did. Everything truly happens for a reason, and even though you may not understand that reason at the moment, God provides the clarity for you to understand it in the future. You just have to be patient with Him and understand He has the best timing!

Fast forward to November 10th, 2009. I was already in my feelings because this was my due date from my second pregnancy the year before. I had gotten into a fight with the roommate I had at the time while living in Georgia. We just couldn't seem to get along, and with all the events I was experiencing that year, I had no room for the extra shit. We fought in our apartment, just her and me. I was on the phone with my best friend Domo when Charlotte came knocking on my door talking to me all crazy. She swung on me first, and it was on from there. By the end of the fight, I was standing behind her with my right arm wrapped around her neck in a way where my wrist was right over her mouth. She bit the hell out of me! I had a bite mark on my wrist and everything.

So, we started fighting again. In the end, I had her in a headlock, and she had my hair. I asked her, *"Are you done?"* and she said, *"Are you?"* I said, *"I'm done, let my hair go!"* and she said, *"I'm done, let my neck go!"* and that was that. I was done after that. I went to call Domo back, and she answered like, *"I'm on my way"* ...I laughed because she was from Chicago, and she stayed ready for whatever. She was and still is my ride-or-die best friend.

In conclusion, 2009 sucked. I had experienced so much sadness, so much devastation that my heart just couldn't handle anymore. I had lost my PaPa, I lost Alex, and I lost my roommate. I lived in Georgia, and I had never felt more alone than I did by the end of 2009. My life was a whirlwind, and everything had hit me like a ton of bricks.

On November 23rd, I wrote:

"Dear Love (my journal,)

I would really like to make this my last journal entry for a looooooong time. I'm tired of being so sad and always writing about bad shit. But I can only write when I'm feeling all emotional. Here I am alone, crying out of control cuz Alex is having a baby on me. I just got done watching Intervention, and it made me feel some type of way. I feel like I need an interventionist. Can you be addicted to love, like being addicted to drugs? I've tried giving my situation to God so many times. I want Him to take all of this pain and anger from me cuz I'm just SO angry that he took my love and my babies from me.

I tried to keep telling myself it wasn't meant for Alex and I to be together and have a child, but my heart just won't accept it. I started back talking to Darius. I don't know if it's cuz I miss him or out of desperation. I'm desperate to get rid of this void Alex left in my life. I always tend to go back to old news. I'm steady settling...I'm too afraid to be alone. To not have someone to call and talk to. Especially now that I live by myself, I feel even more alone now. I love it, but I hate it at the same time. I been having Darius over cuz I don't have no one else...

I want this to be my last entry until I'm happy...I haven't been happy in sooooooo long. Steady holding onto hope, not realizing there wasn't any there. Why is Alex unconsciously putting me through so much? Him not knowing is the worst part. I deserve better. A better friend. A better man. They say that it's when you stop looking that he'll come. So, I'm done looking..."

And just when I thought things couldn't get any worse, just when I thought I had experienced the worst of the worst, *I tested positive for HIV...Oh. Shit.*

"AIDS is real, don't care how you feel. And yes, I want to chill but I gotta wrap it up, I gotta protect us. AIDS is real, don't care how you feel, we already know it kills, So I gotta wrap it up I gotta protect us"

(Lyfe Jennings, Its Real, Lyfe Change)

~ December 21st ~

While searching for love, searching for that, "pick me up," trying to fill this void left in my heart, I contracted HIV. In-between rejecting the feelings I had for Desmond and trying to move on from Alex, I met that guy at the traffic light. There I was, looking the devil himself straight in the eyes, and I did not even know it. But it was not long before I learned that he was a wolf in sheep's clothing.

Aforementioned, he was charming. He was handsome, and he seemed to be well put together. After he had put his hands on me for the first time, I thought I was done with him. And then Papa died, Alex left and was having a baby, and I lived with someone that I could not get along with. I dreaded going to work but dreaded going home even more. In November of 2009, I got a text from Darius just saying what's up. By this time, I had erased his name and number out of my phone, so I had no clue who it was. He apologized for everything he had done to me, for being a jerk, being physically and verbally abusive, and treating me less than I deserved. Of course, I fell for it, and we started talking again. I began to spend a lot of time with him because I was trying to keep my mind off everything else that was going on in my life.

I needed a distraction and what better way than to entertain someone else? After the fight I had with my roommate, my

lymph nodes[9] had swollen badly in my neck. There was an area on the left side of my neck where my lymph node was protruding. It was tender to the touch and it had me concerned, so I scheduled an appointment with my primary care physician. I told the doctor that I had gotten into an altercation and that the girl had bitten me and broke the skin. I do not know why I felt like that mattered at the time, but I did. He felt all the areas housing my lymph nodes. Down the sides of my neck, under my arms, and in my groin area. He had mentioned that all my lymph nodes were swollen, and he was not sure why.

He prescribed me something to get the swelling down and told me to come back in a week. I went back in a week, and the swelling was down on the one that hurt the most, but the rest of my lymph nodes were still swollen. They were not visible by the naked eye, but a physician could most certainly tell by feeling around. My primary care doctor could not figure out what was happening, so he referred me to an **ENT**[10]. The whole time that I was checking in with my doctor, I just thought something happened during the fight that I had. HIV did not cross my mind, not once. When I got to the ENT, I again explained that I had gotten into a fight with my roommate, and everything from the swollen lymph nodes, to the soreness, to the bite mark, seemed to follow that fight. I remember him asking me if I was sexually active. (No idea why that mattered, but okay...)

---

[9] *A small bean-shaped structure that is part of the body's immune system.* Cancer.gov
[10] *Ear, Nose, and Throat doctor.*

He did an assessment, feeling around and asking questions about my overall health. He asked me to open my mouth and looked at the back of my throat. He noticed white spots back there, and I remember him saying it looked like it could be HIV or Lymphoma but that he needed to run tests. He drew several tubes of blood and sent them all to a lab. I do not recall how many, but it had me feeling weak by the time he finished. I looked over at the cart where he sat the tubes, and there looked to be like twenty! The lab results would take a couple of weeks, so he scheduled me for a **biopsy**[11] and advised he would deliver the results when I returned for the surgery. I went home and did all the research I could do on Lymphoma and HIV. The first thing I researched was the symptoms.

I recollect reading about symptoms like fatigue, flu-like symptoms such as fever and chills, muscle aches, and then the most obvious one, swollen lymph nodes. The ONLY symptom I had was the enlarged lymph nodes. I'm thinking, *"Well, if I have to choose, I definitely don't want cancer..."* I mean, imagine having to choose between having HIV and having Lymphoma? Talk about a Catch 22. I was convinced that I had nothing and that I was worrying myself to death for no reason with only experiencing the swollen lymph nodes. The worst part was having to wait for what seemed like forever for the results to come back. My biopsy was

---

[11] *A biopsy is when the doctor takes a tissue sample and sends it off for close examination.*

scheduled for December 21st, 2009, and I was NOT prepared for what was to come that day…

My Godparents took me to the hospital that morning because I was being put under anesthesia and could not operate a vehicle afterward. I checked in at the front desk and was taken back to an operating room. As I sat on the hospital bed waiting, my ENT doctor came in to deliver my lab results as he promised. I sat on the hospital bed with my Godparents sitting kitty-corner from me. My doctor sat next to me, and I remember almost verbatim what he said to me. He said, *"Your tests came back, and there were some positives…"* Almost immediately, my chest was hurting, my armpits were itching, and my palms were sweating. I was so gotdamn nervous! I asked my Godparents to leave the room so he could deliver the news that was about to change my life forever.

I was only twenty-two, and I could tell the doctor was nervous. It was odd because I am sure he has had to do this a million times over, but I'm sure every time is like the first time when you have to deliver bad news. He cleared his throat and proceeded to tell me…

"Your test came back positive for HIV…"

At that point, the word "devastation" would do me no justice. I was mortified. I was so embarrassed, so humiliated. I couldn't even react because I was so dumbfounded. All I remember doing was sitting silently and shaking my head up and down. It was a silent *"Okay, what does that mean? How the hell did I get here?! Who did this to me?!"* I let my Godparents back into the room so I could share the news with them. I still was unsure what this meant for me, but I knew it was serious and that my close family members needed to know. My Godparents didn't know what to say but assured me that they would support me and lend a helping hand and listening ear.

I called my Mom next to tell her because I knew she would be torn to pieces, and I wanted her to hear it from me. I remember my Mom said, *"Uh-uh, this isn't real? Is this real?"* and asking to speak to my Godparents. She then asked them, *"Is she for real? Is this really real?"* That is all she kept asking. She didn't want to believe that her baby girl had HIV, and quite frankly, neither did I. I still hadn't cried yet. I was unaware of what HIV really was, and I was instantly under the impression that I had *AIDS*[12]. It was not until later that I learned that HIV and AIDS were different. The doctor told me I had to contact the people I had sex with for the past twelve months and that if I couldn't carry out that task, there was a way it could be done anonymously.

So, the next person I called was Darius. We were still together at the time, and I was almost certain that he was the reason I was in this predicament. Our past was full of infidelity. He lived a risky lifestyle, and there was no telling what he was doing in the five months that we were apart. I called him, and he was in the streets per usual "making plays."

---

[12] *AIDS is the late stage of HIV and is usually diagnosed when a person's CD4 cells fall below 200 cells per cubic millimeter of blood.* www.hiv.gov

I could tell he was driving because I could barely hear him over the wind in the background as if the windows were down. He rode with the windows down a lot because he was a smoker. I told him I really needed to talk to him about what was going on, and then suddenly, I could hear him clear as day.

I could tell he had rolled the windows up so he could listen to what I had to say because the background noise was no longer there. I asked him to reassure me that he hadn't cheated on me. He confirmed. I asked him had he slept with anyone else unprotected while we were separated, and he said no. So, I swallowed my pride and told him I had just tested positive for HIV. I went on to explain further before he could even respond.

I wanted to get it all out because I was afraid of what he was about to say. I remember talking a lot and him just listening to what I had to say. My palms were sweating, and my voice was shaky. I was a nervous wreck. I couldn't believe I had to have this conversation at twenty-two years old. I remember asking Darius to get tested, and I was genuinely concerned for him and his health. I remember telling him that if his test came back negative, I did not want to continue in a relationship with him because I was afraid I would give it to him and couldn't live with myself if that happened.

As I was going through all this, all I could think about STILL was OTHER PEOPLE. How other people were going to feel and how hurt they were going to be. I was the least concerned about myself. I always worried about others before I worried about myself. I was most concerned about Alex, though. In my mind, I thought, *"It's REALLY over between us now,"* and just feeling so down and overwhelmed with emotions. Darius agreed to get tested, and while agreeing, he scolded me for trying to end the relationship if he didn't have HIV. Because I miscarried the year before, I opted to get tested for HIV and didn't have it then. Then I knew deep down that it was Darius, but I still wanted him to get the test done.

Nonetheless, He repeatedly said, *"That's fucked up. That's fucked up that you expect me to just leave you like that".* And I specifically asked, *"If you test negative, you still wanna be with me???"* and he said, *"Hell yea!"* I remember it like yesterday. It comes to me so vividly because I kept thinking, *"Wow, he really is a ride or die ass dude!" I was winning! Or so I thought…*

Not too long after me, Darius also tested positive for HIV (or so he says). I started using the internet to figure my life out. I looked up how long people with HIV live, their side effects, and how long before I got AIDS and died. It sounds drastic, but it is literally what I spent the next few days doing. I concluded that I would probably get AIDS and die within ten years like my searches turned up…so I planned to get married and have a baby. I kept telling myself that if this was going to kill me, I wanted to leave a legacy, and I wanted to live out my dream of getting married and having one big happy family. My thinking back then was so superficial.

I wish I would have talked to someone and let someone keep me on a better path forward. All I really needed was guidance and a plan. If I could go back, that is one thing I would have done differently. But here I was, making impulsive decisions based strictly on ignorance and emotions. After spilling the beans to my parents, they bought me a flight home to spend the holidays with them. I stayed with my sister that weekend. Everything was different. My family didn't know what to say. They didn't know how to act. My Mom thought my diet needed to change, and almost everyone felt like I couldn't cough around them without them getting the virus.

It felt like the 90's all over again. My Mom and Dad spent their days and nights researching and trying to find things that would comfort me in this time of despair. I laugh about this now, but I remember trying to open a pack of bacon with a knife, and I accidentally cut my finger. It was a tiny cut that drew just a little bit of blood, and my sister freaked out. She's like, *"Can you still cook it?!"* It's funny now, but when it happened, I was just kind of shook.

I honestly wasn't sure if everyone was okay or if I should wear hazmat suits when I came around! It sounds comical, but that is the depth of ignorance we carried at that point in time. I understand now more than ever that education truly is key. The truth was, I could still share drinks. I could still kiss and hug and cough and sweat without spreading HIV to someone else. I learned that along the way, but it was not something I knew when I first tested positive for the virus.

While I was in Chicago, I had spoken to Darius about getting married and starting a family since this virus was my new normal. At this point, he was down for any and everything.

He hadn't gotten his test done yet, but that didn't matter; he was willing and ready to accept me for me and take on these new challenges. I still thought I was winning. I even thought I had finally found the one that was really going to be down to ride forever. I started tracking my ovulation and noted the dates I was likely to get pregnant. I never thought those apps were fully accurate, but I tried it anyway. I flew back to Atlanta a couple of days after Christmas and spent the next few nights with Darius intending to get pregnant.

Music was and still is therapy for me. I looked to music to help me cope with everything. I waited for the night when I was most likely to get pregnant and got really drunk. Darius and I had sex all night long to Trey Songz's *"Ready"* album. This album at this time in our lives was comparable to R. Kelly's *"Twelve Play"* album when our parents were our age. It was one of those albums you could put on repeat and feel the vibes all day and all night. They say many 80's babies were made from R. Kelly jams. Well, many of the 2000's babies were probably made from Jagged Edge and Trey Songz! I can still hear it now… ***"This right here's a panty droppaaaaaa!!!"***

That late-night turned into the early morning. I remember waking up thinking, *"I wonder if it worked?"* I gave myself a couple of weeks and waited for my period to be late before taking a pregnancy test. Before I knew it, I was in the store taking a pregnancy test in the women's bathroom. Yes, I took it INSIDE the store because I could not wait to get home. And what do you know? Within a month of testing positive, I was pregnant...worked like a charm, but what was I REALLY getting myself into? The next few months would be hell on Earth, and this was just the beginning.

"I can't even look you in the face without wanting to slap you, damn I thank God I ain't get that tattoo, you better be glad I ain't have the strap boo, you ain't even worth that trick get at you. Matta fact, trick get at dude. I'm convinced I ain't got shit to ask you. And tell that triflin b**** she can have you, I ain't lookin at you no more, I'm lookin past you. Here we go, here we go again. And you're telling me that she is just a friend, then why she calling you at 3 o'clock in the morning? I can't take this no more"

(Trina feat Kelly Rowland, Here We Go, Still Da Baddest)

∾⊘ **Liar, Liar** ∾⊘

At the end of January, I got a phone call at two in the morning telling me that MY boyfriend had another girlfriend. I was confused and angry, to say the absolute least. First of all, it was 2 a.m. Who thinks rationally when getting woken up out of their sleep by some random chick at that time of the morning? Secondly, I was pregnant, and I had HIV. She had no idea what was coming her way when she decided to make that phone call. Darius happened to be asleep next to me when she rang, and I woke him up and said, *"Your girlfriends on the phone..."* with such a nonchalant attitude. To be honest, I was already exhausted and dealing with so much with just learning that I had HIV, and now I was expecting. He gets on the phone, and he starts cursing this girl out.

I really thought she was just a crazy ex or a "client" who just wanted his attention. He's like, *"Bitch! What the fuck are you doing?! What the fuck is you talkin bout?! You are NOT my Muthafuckin girlfriend!"* He acted very disturbed. Very frustrated that his sleep was interrupted with what he was calling bullshit. He disconnected the call and went into the kitchen to fix a glass of water. I was way too curious about how she got my number and who she was just to let the issue go, so I called her back. This girl starts telling me EVERYTHING about them. She told me how they had been together since our breakup in June and how her one-year-old son calls him, *"Dada."*

She says, *"Jessica, I do not know why he is acting like this! He just dropped me off this morning!"* And I'm like, *"huh?"* She continues to tell me about how he just dropped her off at her place the morning before in *"that green car"* and that he said to her that the green car belonged to one of his "friends." That green car was MY GREEN CAR. It was a '96 Sebring Convertible. My Mom gave it to me when she got a new car so that I could get around and get to my appointments. I had bought a car earlier that year, but I totaled it after only a couple of months, so my Mom was generous enough to give me one with no car note. She ALWAYS took care of me.

Anyway, the girl goes, *"That's your green car??!! We fucked in that car!"* I was sick to my stomach. Legit sick, wanting to puke all over the place sick. I couldn't believe what I was hearing. I walked into the kitchen to confront him, and as he's tipping his glass up to take a drink of that ice-cold water, I flipped the glass up out of his hand and went off on him.

I recalled this night in my journal and wrote:

"You got me walking around with all these diseases and shit and pregnant, and you got the audacity to cheat on me?!" So, I kicked him out at two something in the morning. Didn't give a fuck where he went or who picked his ass up. No phone. Cold as hell. I called one of his family members and said he exposed me to this and that, and I just put his ass

out because his little girlfriend called me...So I told the girl that I was pregnant and that he exposed me to HIV. She starts crying and shit talkin about she got kids to live for...I told him I was getting an abortion. He was PISSED. But I felt like hell, don't think about me and my baby now. You wasn't thinking about us when you were cheating..."

For the next eight months, I had to deal with this girl. I lost count of how many times I waited up for him to come home, and he'd never show because he was with her. She had a nickname for him, and she would post all over her social media whenever they were together. It would be nights that he would promise he would be there for dinner, and he wouldn't show up, and I'd eat all alone. Go to bed alone. And start scrolling through her social media to see, *"Oh, He surprised me and picked me up from work today!"* with the heart emoji's, and I'm just sitting at my dinner table looking ridiculous.

So many times, I wrote that I was done and that I deserved better, and I wasn't settling anymore, but I dealt with him throughout my entire pregnancy. The back and forth became unbearable mentally and emotionally. I wrote about several different times that he made promises and broke them just as quickly as he created them.

I cry when I go back and read things like:

"I'm crying. As usual. Darius was supposed to come over today, but I guess he was so "busy" making plays he couldn't come. I have been calling him all night. No answer. Go figure. I just texted him and said, 'I'm so over you... I'm

going to bed' I just don't get it. I may bitch and nag a lot, and I may have an attitude problem, but I do not mistreat the people I love. I loved Alex so much; Did any and everything for him...I would've much rather dealt with that than deal with what I am dealing with now. HIV. A baby daddy with a girlfriend that has four kids, no place to stay, no money, and no car...and he chose that over me?

I admit I did tell him that it was over and that we would never be together. But hell, He can't do right. I couldn't keep letting him cheat and dog me out. I deserve better, and I know my worth, and I'm worth much more than what he thinks. I was reading the letter Alex wrote to me before I moved here, and I cried. Where did we go wrong? I wasn't supposed to stay here for years. I was supposed to go back and finish school and be with him. MARRY him, have HIS baby. Here I am, pregnant by a man that can't keep his dick in his pants. And Alex is having a little boy with his current girlfriend, and they seem to be so happy. And I'm jealous cuz that should've been us..."

I was so hard on myself. It was impossible to love me back then when I couldn't even love myself. There was another time where Darius was supposed to go to church with me on Easter Sunday, and he promised he was done dealing with that other girl. Well, I had changed my number several times because every time he would sleep with her, she would get my number out of his phone and harass me. It got to a point where HE didn't even have my number. We only talked when I called him restricted, or we communicated via email. That is how bad it was. That is how much I wanted her to leave me alone. But that morning of Easter 2010, I woke up to ten missed calls, and Darius had twenty-nine. All from the same number.

I just knew it wasn't her because he didn't even have my number. To this day, I have no clue how she got that number, but she was pissed off because apparently Darius was supposed to be spending Easter with her. My insecurities let him play the hell out of me. I ended up driving him back to a relative's house where he was living, and the girl was waiting in the parking lot for him. It was beyond insanity to me. I got out of the car and went in behind him, and she yells out the window that I'm a tramp and that "he didn't tell me to go in the fuckin house with him." I just looked back and smiled and kept walking.

At this point, I was becoming numb to it all. I had to, or I was going to drive myself crazy. I had to accept what was and try my best to have a healthy pregnancy. And for that to happen, I had to be on good terms with Darius. I know a part of me felt like I was winning because I was the bigger person. I don't know that winning is a good term to use, but I was certainly being more mature and coming to terms with the fact that I may have to deal with her for a very long time. On May 2nd, 2010, my closest and most favorite cousin was shot and killed. I had just spoken with him days before his death and was ready to tell him that I had HIV and the situation I was now going through with my baby's father.

I wanted his opinion. I wanted to know how having a child changed HIS life, hoping that the same thing would happen after mine was born. It was the end of April, and he answered the phone like he always does … *"Whaddup cuz"*… I was five months pregnant and emotional from all the trauma I was experiencing throughout my pregnancy. He was overprotective, so I never started the conversation with bad news or crying or anything. It was always just, *"Nothing much. Just calling to talk to you…"* and then we would converse about everything. He told me how he knew he had to straighten up after he had his daughter. He wanted to set a good example for her. He wanted to be the father she could look up to and brag about. He was such a good dad. We were only three weeks apart, so we always hung out with each other on our birthdays.

During this particular conversation, he advised me to give my baby's father time. He told me sometimes kids do change a person, but sometimes they don't. He said, either way, I needed to be strong for my baby. I wanted so bad to tell him I had contracted HIV, but I couldn't fix my mouth to deliver the news. Instead, I invited him to my coed baby shower and threatened that he better be there, or I was going to kick his ass. He said he wouldn't miss it. It was planned for May 22nd in my hometown. I remember him saying, *"This my baby momma calling me now, I'm gonna call you right back,"*….and he never called back. It was okay because he did that to me all the time. But this time, it would be the last conversation I ever had with him. A couple of days later, I had woken up to missed calls from another close cousin and from a close friend I had at the time.

I called my cousin back first because she rarely called me, so I knew it was serious. In calling her back, I get a text from my friend saying, *"Please tell me it ain't true?"* and I was just utterly confused. My cousin picks up, and she goes, *"Are you okay, cuz? You okay?"* And at this point, I am just like, *"WHAT THE HELL IS GOING ON?!!!"* Sydney texted me, and you called me a few times, and I don't even know what anyone is talking about!"* And she said, *"Cameron was shot, and he died this morning..."* I freaking lost it. I kept denying that it was true because I had just talked to him a couple of days before, and he said he would call me back. We both just cried. He died from gunshot wounds at only twenty-two years old.

My twin brother and Cameron were extremely close, and his death was even more devastating for my twin. I couldn't believe it. He wasn't going to be here to meet my baby. He wasn't going to be here to congratulate me at the baby shower and talk his shit and crack his jokes. I took this time to reach out to Alex's mom and let her know that I had tested positive and that he should get tested. I couldn't dare reach out to Alex and tell him myself. I was deathly afraid of how he was going to react and what he was going to say. I knew his mom could say it to him in a way that wouldn't cause panic or anger, so I asked her to tell him. She was sad for me. She was devastated, but she was supportive, and she was encouraging. She loved me like her own daughter back then and her and I are still very close today.

I just balled when I told her, and I said, *"If Alex and I would've just worked it out, I wouldn't be here!"* I was angry with the world, and I couldn't handle the grief along with what I was already dealing with. I was looking for a scapegoat, but there was none in sight. People grieve differently. And there is no standard to grieving. Some people pick up bad habits like drugs and alcohol due to grief or family loss. Some people write music or poetry or books. Some people start experiencing depression and become withdrawn. There are so many ways to grieve, and my way at this point in my life was finding comfort.

I went straight to Darius to be consoled. I went to him to be held and to cry on his shoulder. This time though, Darius didn't provide much solace, but I took what I could get. I spent the night with him that night and went back to my apartment the next day and grieved at home. I was so alone. I was pregnant, alone, and angry. In my head, I was stuck with him because no one wanted someone pregnant with HIV. So, for the next four or five months, I was going to have to suffer through. The weekend after his death, Darius decided he would go to a bar and play pool. I expected him to meet up with friends and maybe have a few drinks and head back home.

However, when I talked to him, he said he was alone. So, me knowing him and knowing that he still hadn't let that other girl go, I checked her social media. Sure enough, her status says she was going to go play pool and drink with her "Baby Daddy." The next day, I call him and completely spazzed on him. He was such a liar when it came to her. He wouldn't answer his phone some nights all night long and just swear he was asleep, or he didn't hear his phone when the entire time it was because he was sleeping with her. I was sick of being lied to and being put on the back burner for her.

On June 23rd, I wrote:

"Well...me and Darius are over. It's pretty much official. This is the second time he has dropped me like a bad habit to go back to that girl. Where the hell did all my pride and morals go? How did he even get another chance to do this to me? A week ago, he texted me and said he felt we could work on us. Two days ago, he said he didn't want to hurt me anymore, and he loves me, and he's happy with me. And then yesterday he's back with Ol' girl, and he's not ready for a relationship with me...I can't let him keep doing this to me. Play with me like a doll and put me back on the shelf. I can't believe he did it AGAIN..."

He only did it again because I let him. And as long as I let him continue to mistreat me, he wasn't going to stop. I knew this in my head, but my heart couldn't let him go. I didn't want to be alone raising a child. I didn't want to be a single mother before my child was even here. I didn't want to be that stereotypical black woman, that "bitter baby momma." But what was I going to do? I wanted something that he clearly didn't want. But at the time, I wasn't strong enough to walk away….so I stayed. Until one day, I had enough. At the end of July, Darius and I had gone to register for the second baby shower I had in Atlanta. He had to leave to take that other girl's son home.

He was supposed to come back, but of course, he never showed. I put my phone on silent that night and went to sleep. I woke up at 6 a.m. to a text that said, *"Me bitch that's who"*…I was confused because the last thing I had sent to his phone was about my car. I called her, and I immediately start cussing her out! Darius and I were over, and I made it very clear to him AND her, so I wasn't sure why she was calling me and harassing me. I was 33 weeks pregnant and at risk of preterm labor if I continued to let her rile me up. So, I called the police on her and filed a harassment report.

The officer came to my apartment, and she happened to still be calling when he showed up. He answered my phone and told her she needed to stop calling, or she was going to be in trouble. After the officer left, she called fourteen more times. After calling fourteen times, she sent another text saying, *"Bitch, I hope you die having that baby, you diseased whore."* So, I called the officer back and added that to the report. This time, he ran her info, and she had a failure to appear warrant. It was the same warrant that Darius had, landing him in jail that night. That is why she was blowing me up. They had gotten drunk and got into a fight, and the police were called for them disturbing the peace. Darius had warrants, so they took him to jail, and she used that as an opportune time to harass me.

One week into being locked up, he wrote me a letter. It said:

"Wassup baby? First, let me start off with I fucked up hella hella hella bad, and I did you hella wrong, and again I'm hella sorry!! And I mean it for real, ma. I understand something this deep will never just go away...I don't know what to tell you on paper to make you really see and understand that I'm so done with that girl for good...There's death with her and life without her for real...Whatever I have to do to show you she's dead to me I will..."

I had enough of that girl. I had enough of the two together. My birthday weekend came, and Darius was still in jail from the incident. I was 36 weeks, and I wasn't sure he would be out in time to see our child born. I went and took maternity pictures on my birthday to keep my mind off the position I was in. I just wanted to feel pretty for ONE day. I wanted to feel confident, and I did just that. I had gone to the mall and got a full application of makeup done. The store I went to had a bunch of makeup counters and perfume counters with all different brands. I had three different changes of clothes too. I was making my twenty-third birthday all about me, unapologetically. They turned out to be beautiful pictures.

I was on my way to restoring my confidence and being a better me. Darius was trying his hardest to jeopardize that by making broken promises through his jail letters.

On August 20th, 2010, he wrote:

"I guess this is my thank you letter. Cause I really do thank you for forgiving me and giving me another chance to bring back Darius and to show you my real heart, and my real love, my real sweet and caring self. I definitely didn't mean to nor wanted to hurt you like I did...I don't want to keep talking about what I'm gonna do when I get home. I just want to do it! You feel me! I can write about it all day, every day, but as we know, actions speak louder than these words on these papers..."

In another letter, he wrote:

"I want you and need you in my life so bad, but I'm scared, ya know. I know I'm not gonna cheat on you. I'm so done. I just want one. I learned my lesson, dead ass. I'm not gonna lie anymore...I'm done with drinking and smoking...me putting my hands on you is done as well...I promise to stay away from that girl for good. I got it in my head that her kid is not mine. I have one and only one, and that's how it will stay..."

He was promising to be a better man and a better father for his child and me. Although I was physically and emotionally drained, I STILL wasn't strong enough to walk away from the relationship. I let his letters get to me over time, and I was convinced we would be a family again when he got out of jail. Talk about toxic. He said he would do anything to show me that he's for real this time and that he's ready to change for his child and me. He wrote a letter to my parents asking for their forgiveness. He even asked me to marry him! He apologized for "opening a new door without closing the old one," and promised things would be different. I fell for it...I fell for all of it... and to no one's surprise, **it was all lies.**

"You think you got the best of me. Think you've had the last laugh? Bet you think that everything good is gone. Think you left me broken down, think that'd I'd come running back, baby you don't know me cuz you're dead wrong. What doesn't kill you makes you stronger"

(Kelly Clarkson, Stronger (What Doesn't Kill You))

❧ **Daddy, He Knew...** ☙

On September 15th, I had my firstborn baby. She was right on time despite all the circumstances I went through to get her here. She was 7 pounds, 1 oz. My Mom said, *"Dang Jessie! You had a Kindergartener!"* I still laugh at that part of the video when I watch her being born. Back then, you could record it without fear of the footage being used against the doctor if something went wrong. A lot of doctors don't allow recording anymore. If you're wondering if Darius was present, he was. He had gotten out of jail on September 13th. I purposely scheduled my induction to take place after his court date because I really wanted him to be there. He went to court on the 13th and got released that night.

I went into the hospital the night of the 14th. I was 39 weeks. My doctor didn't want me to go to 40 weeks because it was a high-risk pregnancy due to me having HIV (even though my viral load was undetectable.) Darius got out and stayed the first night in my apartment. He promised to be present in the letters, be faithful, and never contact that girl again. The doctor's appointment I had the week before then showed that I was not **dilated**[13] at all, so I knew my daughter was not going to come on her own. Well, Darius and I had sex the first night he was out, and when I went

---

[13] *make or become wider, larger, or more open.* Oxford Languages

73

into the hospital the next night, I was 1 cm dilated. I went in at about 8:30 that night, and eventually, they gave me a medication to help induce labor.

Once labor started, I got medication for the pain, and when the contractions became more consistent and more intense, they gave me an epidural. All I remember after that is falling asleep, and I woke up vomiting. As I was puking, my water broke, and the nurses rushed in and told me to get ready to push. I was in labor for a total of five hours. Four pushes later, she was here.

They put her on an oral medication they called **AZT**[14]. She was on AZT for her first six weeks of life. She was tested within a few hours and then twice more after that by the time she was six months old. After her final test was done and came back negative, she didn't have to have any more tests done. I was blessed that I did not pass it to my newborn, which was one of my biggest fears. I was about to start this journey of being a new mom while still dealing with accepting the fact that I had HIV.

I was on the longest, most tumultuous emotional rollercoaster. It seemed like it was never going to end. I was not very educated on **postpartum depression**[15] until later, after I had other kids. I realize now how much I was suffering back then, and I was suffering in silence. I had an

---

[14] *Zidovudine. An antiretroviral medication that helps prevent the baby from getting HIV.*

[15] *Also called PPD, is a medical condition that many women get after having a baby. It's strong feelings of sadness, anxiety (worry), and tiredness that last for a long time after giving birth.* Marchofdimes.org

inkling that Darius was still talking to Ol' girl, but I was too consumed in other things to investigate. If you go looking for it, chances are you will find it, so this time I didn't look for it.

I tried just to be happy with our family and pray that things would just come together. I had a nice apartment in Kennesaw, GA, but I wanted a two-bedroom that I could afford on my own because Darius wasn't reliable. We ended up moving to Canton, GA, to a two-bedroom apartment on the third floor. To this day, I REFUSE to ever live on the third floor of an apartment ever again. I'd end up having to truck groceries and a newborn up and down two flights of stairs for longer than I could bear! Anyhow, it didn't take long before his phone was going off at all hours of the night. He rarely ever heard his phone at night. One night, his messages were going off at 2 a.m., and I couldn't help but read them this time. It was from a different chick who was apparently just friends with him.

The messages talked about how she wanted to *"Fuck him and sit on his face."* But the message that got me fired up was her telling him she missed my baby. One could not even IMAGINE the fury that was flowing through my body when I saw that text. I couldn't believe that not only was he STILL cheating, but he was taking my baby over to another woman's house. My blood was boiling. I woke him up out of his sleep and got very, very physical with him. I was punching, screaming, and crying. He called for a ride and ended up leaving for a couple of days. I have no idea where he went, and I could give a fuck less. I just wanted him out of my life for good. My Godparents owned a transportation business at the time, and their holiday party was approaching.

Darius and I were not together but were trying to make the best of the situation. I was working a late shift (5 p.m. to 2 a.m.), so I needed him at my house to help me with my baby. We tried to make it work. We attended the party at an elegant hotel. There was food and music and an open bar. The open bar was trouble for anyone who didn't know their drinking limit. Darius got drunk, and we ended up arguing because I felt as if he was embarrassing me. He was laughing at stuff that, to me, wasn't funny and making inappropriate jokes. We were on the fourth floor of the hotel after the party hanging with my Godparents.

As we left their room to head to the car, I stated that he was embarrassing while walking down the hallway. I don't know if that was a trigger for him, but he went into this rage that reminded me of the first time he had ever put his hands on me. I remember precisely what coat and shoes I had on that night because one shoe was missing, and my coat had the buttons ripped off by the end of the night. We ended up in the elevator, and he grabbed me by the collar of my coat and damn near lifted me off my feet. He was looking me dead in my face, and I told him he was hurting me, but it was like he was looking right through me.

His eyes looked like black holes, and his face was beet red. He was angry, to say the very least. I kept hitting the elevator buttons, trying to get off on the first floor where the lobby was. I remember the elevator doors opening a couple of times, but no one was waiting on them. The doors would close, and there I was stuck again, tussling with him. When it finally stopped on the first floor, he hooked his arms under mine and carried me out of the elevator. I was screaming and crying, and there were three older white men in the lobby that came to my rescue. Darius took off in my car, and the hotel lobby workers called the police.

The police showed up and took a police report. They got my information on the vehicle to run the plates and try to track him down. I only had one shoe on, and all the buttons were ripped off my coat. It was a two-hundred-dollar coat with huge ruffles around the collar. It was a pretty candy apple red, knee-length peacoat. I loved that coat! Anyway, the officer asked, *"Did that happen as a result of the altercation.?"* I stated, *"Yes."* I had scratches on my face and my neck. He asked about those as well and took notes as I explained what had happened. I was so embarrassed! I worried about our baby because she was at home with a relative of his. I called her as soon as I got the chance to tell her not to let Darius take her with him because he was drunk and raging out of control.

The officers were able to track him down and pulled him over. I remember the officer calling me after they caught him and told me he was doing 95 mph when the speed limit was 75. He was calling me while speeding, telling me he was trying to flip the car and that he wanted to kill himself.

I recounted every single moment of this in my journal. It was one of the worst nights ever. On December 12th, 2010, he went back to jail. Here we go again. This time I had an almost three-month-old baby, and I had no idea who would be able to watch her while I was working nights. I only had a couple of days to figure it out, seeing that I had to return to work.

I called Darius's family member and asked him to stay with us for a little while and help me with the baby. He didn't mind because he wasn't in the best living situation anyway. That settled one worry, but there was plenty more where that came from.

Aforementioned, when I'm grieving or feeling over-whelmed with emotions, I tend to go back to the last person I felt safe with. So, guess who I called? By April of 2011, I was back to calling Alex. Lord knows I was setting myself up for failure time after time, but yet and still, I continued to reach out and not accept the fact that he wanted nothing to do with me and that he was happy.

On April 25th, 2011, I wrote:

"…I just basically let the cat out the bag and opened up and told him I wasn't over him although I tried to be. I told him a part of me wanted to say fuck it, but another part wanted him back and never let go. I told him how I always said maybe a few years from then (when we broke up) it'll all work out, and here we are a few years later, and I'm still not over him…So, I'm like I just need you to answer this one thing, 'Are we over forever?' And he said he couldn't answer

that; he's not in control of it. As much as he would like to think he is. So, I continued to pour out my heart, and when I said I thought I was the reason he changed his number, his response was this...

'Naw, I just been dealin with a lot... which I know you can relate. I'm not gonna say I don't think about you sometimes cuz I do...a part of me does miss you, and we have grown in more ways than one. I'm not gonna say we will never be together ever again, but I won't tell you we will. I don't wanna set you up to let you down, and yes, I sort of miss you...lol. Don't tell nobody I said that.'

So, I finally got answers. It took three years but hey, better late than never."

Ugh. I was so toxic. And I mean that in the humblest way. Sometimes, you just must admit when you were once that bad apple! I mean, who puts someone in that position? Why did I even ask him that question? I was drowning in grief and anger and confused as to what purpose I was serving anymore. Here I am, a single mother with HIV and a seven-month-old baby. By this time, my twin, his wife, and stepdaughter at the time moved to Georgia to help me with my daughter. Darius's family member ended up moving out, so it was just us. My twin and his wife were a lot of help, but his wife and I weren't getting along, and she ended up moving to Tennessee. My brother stayed just a little while longer, and then he ended up leaving too.

So, Darius's family member was back and forth at my place. When I had to work, he would come over and keep the baby for me. He was such a blessing to us. I was grateful to still have him through it all. However, devastation came knocking at my door once again. On June 5th, 2011, my whole viewpoint on life (and people) changed.

For some reason, I woke up out of my sleep at like 3:45 that morning. I was up like it was 3:00 in the afternoon, all wide-eyed and bushy tailed. I took a sleeping pill to fall back asleep, and while that was kicking in, I was up talking to Darius's family member. We were just chopping it up, having a general conversation about life.

I was telling him how done I was with Darius, and he said, *"For good? Like y'all will never ever be together?"* and I said, *"Yes."* I explained that I felt he was immature and that he wasn't really trying to be in his daughter's life because of the stupid decisions he made that jeopardized his being there for her. One stupid decision I brought up was that he wasn't taking meds. At this point, Darius knew he had HIV, and I had never seen him take anything to help control the virus. I'm telling this to his family, and he gets the craziest look on his face. He looked puzzled. Like I said something that completely took him by surprise.

He was under the impression that Darius was taking medication to help suppress the virus. I said, *"No, he's not on any medication."* and the family member said, *"Yes, he is?"* Again, trying to sound confident but still sounding slightly perplexed. I go on to tell him that I had never seen him take anything, and it would be hard for me to miss seeing that since we were living together. So, his family member says, *"Well, he probably hasn't taken it in a minute, since he was like 17 or 18, but he used to take like five pills a day. He had a Monday thru Sunday pillbox and everything that he used to carry. But for some reason, he just stopped taking it."*

To say I was livid would be doing my feelings a serious injustice. I was outraged! I'm getting loud and telling him how Darius said to me that he did not know he had HIV until recently. The look on his face after THAT statement was more like, *"Huh?"* He couldn't' believe it. He looked astonished, and then he smacked his lips so hard and said, *"Man, that motherfucker knew. He was born with it. His Mom had it."* His family member thought I knew all this already since we had been together so long. In his mind, it made sense for me to know, but I had no clue. I couldn't do anything but sit there and look stupid. I couldn't believe it. I was devastated all over again.

I was appalled. Not to mention, sad and pissed off that not only did he knowingly expose ME to HIV, but he exposed other women to it as well, and they had no idea. Darius was still in jail for domestic battery and a **DUI**[16] he received after the holiday party, so I couldn't take my anger out on him. I obviously couldn't sleep after that conversation, so around 6:30 a.m., I called my Dad. My Dad and I have always been remarkably close, and he always had the best advice and a cool head. He was always the person to help me be rational.

---

[16] *Driving under the influence of alcohol or drugs*

I wanted to hurt something or someone, and I did not know how to channel the anger that had just built up in me. I was surprised he answered because it was actually 5:30 a.m. his time, and I knew he was asleep. He always answered for me no matter what time it was. He picks up, and I just start bawling my eyes out. All I could get out of my mouth was, *"He knew Daddy! He knew! He knew the whole time!"* My Dad just let me cry. He started to talk to me about the kinds of people in this world and explained that some people just do not give a fuck about me. Regardless of how much I give, how kind I am, how good I treat them, they are about self, and nothing else matters. From that point on, I didn't put anything past anybody, and trust was no longer a part of my vocabulary. From now on, it was my baby and me against the world. *I can't believe he was born with HIV and didn't tell me...*

"I don't want to forget the present is a gift, and I don't wanna take for granted the time you may have here with me. Cuz Lord only knows another day here's not really guaranteed. So, every time you hold me, hold me like this is the last time. Every time you kiss me, kiss me like you'll never see me again"

(Alicia Keys, Like You'll Never See Me Again, As I Am)

∽ **Seeking Solace Part 1** ∽

I spent the next six to seven years seeking **solace**[17]. I had no idea where I was going to find it, but I was desperately looking. I made a decision based on emotions and quit my job after finding out he was born with HIV. I needed to be closer to home. I wanted my Mom. I wanted to be around my immediate family for more emotional support. I went into my job late the day after finding out about Darius's status, and my manager told me he recommended me for termination. I knew I was on a written already because there were plenty of times I was late or couldn't show because of my relationship issues.

I didn't have the energy or mental capacity to argue with him, so I quit. I turned in a one-day notice and quit. I called my parents and told them I got laid off because otherwise, they wouldn't let me move back home with them. Plus, they know I make impulse decisions, and they would have been very upset to find out that I quit because I was about to get fired anyway. They would have tried to convince me to stay and get another job or something, and I was beyond ready to leave. I remember Darius was still calling me from jail and had no idea that his family member accidentally ratted him out.

---

[17] *Comfort or consolation in a time of distress or sadness.* Dictionary.com

He called me the day after I found out, **and I asked him did he know way before 2010 that he had HIV**. He played so stupidly with me. I said, *"I heard you were born with the shit!"* And he starts going off on me! He's asking me what the fuck am I talking about and telling me he's only known as long I have known. He was lying, but I couldn't tell him who told me because I didn't want to damage their relationship. I was looking out for his family member, not for him. So, I got smart. I looked up the charges for knowingly exposing someone to HIV/ knowingly infecting someone, and I used that as leverage.

I told him if he didn't tell me the truth, I would get a lawyer and "sue the shit" out of him. So, he confessed. He went on to say he doesn't like to talk about it, and he doesn't like to speak about his Mom. *"How can you be so damn selfish?!!!!"* I was screaming on the phone, talking to him pacing the parking lot of my apartment complex. I could not believe he did this to me, and knowingly! Since he was calling from jail, our time was limited. So, when the call hung up, I called a relative of his. I just knew she knew. She picks up, and I immediately ask her, *"How long has Darius had HIV?!!!!"*

I was confident in my question. I was stern, and I didn't hesitate. I wasn't asking *IF* he had it, but I indicated that I had found something out, and I was basically seeing if she would confirm. Her response to me after moments of silence was, *"I'm gonna let him tell you that..."* I was infuriated! Did she *really* think he would grow a conscious and tell me? I had been living with HIV for eighteen months, and not one time did ANYBODY ever suggest that he had something I should know about. She proceeds to ask me can she call me back after the basketball game. She had friends over and, *"Couldn't talk about this right now."* I just hung up on her and stormed back into the house.

My mind was going a million miles a minute. I was thinking about all the time I had spent with him and his family. I was thinking about the drama and trauma I experienced during my entire pregnancy. I thought about how he told other women that I exposed HIM HIV, knowing he knew from day one. I thought about how shocked and surprised he acted when I told him I had HIV in the first place. I couldn't fathom it all. I was having a meltdown with no one there to console me. I spent the next few years trying to find comfort in my situation. I looked for a scapegoat. I looked for closure. I looked for an apology. I moved back in with my Mom for a little while and decided to go back to college and finish my degree.

In seeking solace, I had to keep my mind busy. Idle time for me was dangerous. It allowed my mind to wander places I never wanted to go again. While living with my Mom, I was back on my old stomping grounds. I was back around people who supported me, and people I grew up with that knew me. I was not open to telling many people I had HIV, but I did tell my best friend at the time. I should've known that I would regret that based on our history, but again, I just wanted comfort. I needed someone to remind me that everything was going to be okay, and she gave me that, even if it only lasted a short while. A childhood friend of mine named Isaiah messaged me on social media not too long after moving back to Illinois. He was trying to see me and spend time with me.

I knew I wasn't emotionally available, but I also knew that I wanted to feel loved again. I needed to feel wanted, and I missed having the affection that comes with being in a relationship (a good one, at least.) I kept denying him the opportunity and tried to convince myself that I wanted no parts of being with someone from my hometown. But he was persistent, and he was not letting up. So, I agreed to spend some time with him. Well, one thing lead to another, and before I knew it, I had a boyfriend. I was already planning to return to college and finish the degree I left behind when I moved to Georgia. I got into that relationship, and he moved back to southern Illinois with my daughter and me.

He was a sweet guy, and he had children, and he was really good with my daughter. He knew me before I had HIV, so when I explained my situation to him, he was very understanding and was more than willing to accept me for me. Here I was once again trying to fill a void that would take a lot more than a good boyfriend to fill. But at the time, no one could tell me anything. I was marching to the beat of my own drum. We moved from northern Illinois to southern Illinois at the end of 2011 and started our life together. It was a change of scenery for him, and I was excited to finish what I had started in 2005.

I should have known it wasn't going to be that easy. As soon as we got settled, the messages came. The private messages on his social media, the text messages from people close to him asking him if he knew I had HIV. I remember reading one message that said, *"I know you don't know me like that, but I know Jessica Glaspie, and I know she has AIDS,...And she's telling people."*

I laughed because, number one, I didn't have AIDS. I had HIV[18].

Number two, I'm telling people? I had only told a select few, and I should have known news like that would spread like wildfire in a small town like Zion. You would think they would appreciate me telling people instead of putting people in the position that someone else put me in. The text messages came from people from different areas of his life, but one of them read, *"I heard about your girl...So you got it too?"* It was mind-boggling how much he was getting harassed for being with someone who had HIV. People needed to get educated and get themselves some business because we were going to make it work, and they were going to have to accept that. The first semester back was rough.

---

[18] *(Human immunodeficiency virus) is a virus that attacks the body's immune system. If HIV is not treated, it can lead to <u>AIDS</u>. Acquired immunodeficiency syndrome.* www.cdc.gov

I had an eighteen-month-old, and we moved into a place with nothing. We requested a furnished apartment (we were living on the college campus in family housing, so we had a two-bedroom apartment,) but the furniture wasn't there yet because we moved in early. The floors were hard tile floors, and it was December, so they were cold. We bought two air mattresses and slept that way for a few weeks until we got furniture. I was kind of embarrassed, but him? He didn't mind one bit. He adjusted very well to his environment. Come January of 2012, we had furniture, and I was ready to start my classes. I was looking for work, but we were living off refund checks until I got something. I finally got a job in March, working for a large retailer.

I felt like I was starting to get the consolation I was looking for. I had a good man, I had my daughter, and now I had a job…And then I found out I was expecting my second child. That was definitely not part of the plan. My first thought was my parents are going to be PISSED! And my second thought was abortion. I barely had a two-year-old, and here I was about to bring another baby into the world. I was never *FOR* abortions, so I do not judge anyone that is, but I made my bed, so I should lie in it, right? After talking it over with my NEW baby's father, we decided we were going to terminate the pregnancy. I had just gotten back into school, and I was still dealing with so many other issues. I did not want to bring a child into my chaos.

So, we went to an abortion clinic in Missouri. We were considered the St. Louis Metropolitan area since we were so close to St. Louis, and that is why we ended up in Missouri. Any who, we set an appointment, and when we arrived, we signed in and took a seat. I kept asking him if he was sure he wanted to do this, and he was sure, but I was starting to feel uncertainty. They took me to the back and gave me an ultrasound to see how far along I was. I was eleven weeks. I recall moving step-to-step. Like, step one was an Ultrasound, step two was something else, and so on and so forth.

I got to the end, and a worker sat me down and asked me if I knew there were other alternatives to abortion. I was confused as to why this was the last step of the process. At this point, aren't people already sure that this is what they want to do? I assured her that I wanted the abortion. At the time, the state of Missouri made you wait 24 hours after your first appointment to get the procedure done. I went home and slept on the idea, and the next day I didn't go back. I had a change of heart. Now I understand why they ask you that question at the end. Isaiah wasn't very excited about it, and I knew this would be a challenge with already having a two-year-old, but I didn't think it was fair to abort the baby. I was due December 29th, which was perfect timing for school. I planned it all out. I would be on Christmas break. I could finish the Summer and Fall semester and just take off the Spring semester after I had the baby.

My relationship was volatile. I was emotionally unstable, and I should have never jumped into the relationship so fast.

But in looking for comfort and acceptance, I just wanted it to be so bad that I didn't see how much this wasn't working for us. I was defensive, I was insecure, and I was abusive. Any small thing he did that I felt was wrong or disrespectful would set me off. If we argued and he got in my face, I would feel provoked and hit him. I was on edge all the time. I always felt threatened and couldn't shake my urge to hit something when I was mad. I was triggered by being in enclosed spaces and hearing doors or cabinets slam. When I started to go to therapy for the first time, my therapist diagnosed me with **PTSD**[19].

Because of my elevator experience, I was automatically triggered by being in small spaces with closed doors. I would just lash out and start punching and kicking and fighting my way out of the room. It could be a bedroom, bathroom, anything. I had no business being in a relationship with all the healing I needed to do. And not only was I in a relationship, but I was also having a baby. My poor boyfriend had such damaged goods, and he did not know how to handle it. My son decided to come way sooner than December 29th. Instead of having a Christmas baby, I had him before Thanksgiving.

I had him at 32 weeks. Because he was a preemie, he had to stay in the **NICU**[20] for about one month. He hadn't developed the ability to suck and swallow by 32 weeks, so he couldn't come home until he could take a full bottle.

---

[19] *(Posttraumatic stress disorder.*
[20] *Neonatal intensive care unit*

Imagine having to visit your baby that YOU BIRTHED in the hospital. Imagine not being able to hold him or her and reaching your hands into two small holes to interact with your child. What kind of solace was this?!!! I was feeling worse now than I did before I got there. The depression was real, and my relationship was going to shit.

After I was able to bring him home, I was overwhelmed. He ate every three hours in the NICU, and he stayed on that feeding schedule for about six or seven months. I was up around the clock either feeding him, working, or going to school. It took a significant toll on my mental health, and I just couldn't do it anymore. One night, Isaiah came home after being out for a few hours, and he was supposed to bring something I needed for the baby. But he came home with nothing. So, I got upset, and we started arguing. I was overtired and was not in the mood to argue, so I called my best friend Tiffany and asked if we could come to stay at her house.

Of course, She complied. As I'm packing our stuff, he comes up behind me and says, *"So you finna leave?!"* I ignored him and continued to pack our things, and the arguing continued. I think about it now, and I shake my head because it was just crazy for us to be acting like that. It was crazy to act like that, but we were young, and we were still learning how to cope and parent. The neighbor called the police about a noise complaint. They showed up and asked me if I wanted him to leave, and I said, *"No."* and that my kids and I would go instead. When they left, we started fighting again, and the neighbor calls the police AGAIN. This time he told them it sounded like we were "rearranging furniture."

They came back, and he went to jail. He was released the next day, and we weren't supposed to have contact with each other for 72 hours. They were threatening to kick me out of housing, and I could NOT afford to get kicked out of school. Due to us fighting in the home with children present, the police contacted **DCFS**[21]. I had to meet with them once a week for six months or until they felt I was no longer endangering my children's welfare. That was one of my biggest regrets. I never gave myself time to heal my wounds before trying to move on. I was no good for myself, so there was no way I could be right for someone else.

He was also dealing with past relationships; he and I together was yet again a perfect storm. Seeking solace had gotten me into some shit that was taking forever to get out of. At this point, I decided I just wanted to be by myself and continue going to therapy and give myself time to heal. He and I have a good relationship now, and I really don't think that would be possible had we not gone through this particular storm. It was most certainly a lesson learned, but that was just the beginning of what was to come.

---

[21] *Department of children and family services.*

I don't wanna be your ex
We way too good at being friends
Can we still hangout
On the low, get wild
I don't wanna be your, I don't wanna be
your Ex

(Kiana Lede, Ex)

∼⌒ **Seeking Solace Part 2** ⌒∼

When that relationship ended, my son was only four months old. Now, I was a college student with two children and a single mom. We had a hard time getting along for some years. We both had a lot of growing up to do when it came to parenting. He took on raising my daughter because her Dad was not a constant in her life. I wanted him to be more present and to spend more time, but after trying for so long, I just gave up and took what I could get as far as time went. I was grateful that he still considered my daughter to be his, and he is still a part of her life today.

There were some days I had to take my newborn to class with me. He would get chronic ear infections and had stomach problems from being a preemie. As a result, he would often spike fevers and be sent home from daycare. At first, I would be embarrassed having to bring a baby to class, but with my 10K in room and board and tuition and fees, I dared someone say something. Nowadays, I have seen teachers make the news for carrying babies while teaching and trying to calm their cries. When I brought my baby boy to class, the stares I got had me ready to pack up and leave. But I knew what I was there to do, so failing was not an option whether I had a baby in tow or not. After he and I broke up, guess who I called? Yep, Alex again. I was back at the school where I had met him, so I couldn't help but to reach out. Plus, now he was closer. When I say he was my comfort zone, that's exactly what it was for me. But the solace that I was finding in him, he wasn't finding in me, and it broke my heart every. single. time.

I couldn't figure it out and the rejection was killing me. He didn't answer but he ended up reaching back out to me. He made small talk by congratulating me on my son's birth.

The conversation took off from there. I wrote:

"I don't think I'll EVER love another man like I loved him. Shit is crazy. I hope to one day, but no luck so far." I think the thing that kept me so involved with Alex was the fact that we never fought and rarely argued. He was easy to talk to and slow to anger. When we separated, I had been looking for love in all the wrong places ever since.

I tried to move on from him once again, but the guys I was running into weren't giving me the feels. This quest for consolation was getting to be exhausting. I talked to a guy for a few months day in and day out only to find out he was married! He lied to me and told me he was divorced, but he wasn't and ended up back with his wife. Then, I gave an old boo a try. He was someone I had strong feelings for when I was in college, the first go-round in 2006. I really liked him, but he was in love with his high school sweetheart. He and I were on and off (mostly off,) and then in 2014, I asked him if he ever thought we could be something serious.

I remember him being completely honest and telling me he wanted to marry his high school sweetheart. Before I knew it, he was engaged to be married. I was just like, *"Welp; there goes that idea..."* I was desperate for love and I wanted confirmation that I was still worth something. I felt so empty. So, back to Alex I go! We kind of rekindled and started talking again and spending a little time with each other. At this point, he had accepted my status and was coming around more. I know you're probably thinking, *"Gotdamn!!!! How many times is she gonna go back???"* I didn't want anyone else in the world but him.

And every time a relationship failed, he was my go-to. I knew he didn't want to be with me, but I think he couldn't dare reject me or tell me no because of what I was going through. I was always within arm's reach of him. And I allowed it to be that way for a very long time...I felt like dirt on the bottom of someone's shoe. I had gone back to school because I needed to find a way to make it through. I needed to keep busy to stay away from having that idle mind. Not only that, but I also wanted to show that I wasn't just a black girl with kids and HIV. **I was an EDUCATED black WOMAN with kids and HIV.**

My degree was unfinished business. I felt like if I didn't finish school, I would have absolutely nothing to offer someone. My way of thinking kept me grounded back then, but it destroyed my self-esteem in the process. I was still looking for the light at the end of the tunnel, and to me, that light was nowhere in sight. I graduated in 2015 and got my degree in Business Management. My graduation was AMAZING. I had family and friends from near and far attend. They were so proud of me for completing my degree in spite of all the speed bumps I hit along the road.

My Mom and Dad were especially excited as I was the first one of my siblings to obtain a degree. I don't think anyone expected me to finish under the circumstances. My Godparents flew from Atlanta to be there. They had literally been there since day one…literally. So, they understood the emotions I felt when I walked that stage. Alex's parents attended my graduation as well. They were super proud of me for pushing through. I had a graduation dinner afterward, and everyone was there…except Alex. He says I didn't personally invite him, so he didn't come, but at this point, I'm pretty sure he was just over me and sick of my shit (I mean, wouldn't you be?)

I felt accomplished, but I still felt empty. I always felt like something was missing, but I couldn't figure out what that something was. For a long time, I felt like Alex was that "something," and it took all of this plus more for me to realize he was not my missing piece. Since we were still on good terms (even after graduation.) I even tried to get him to move with me, but that was a hard no. He was way too involved with his son and wouldn't dare be that far away from him. I took a job close to my parents right after college and relocated. In June of that year, I started working my first full-time "big girl" corporate position.

I was in an entry-level Supply Chain job. Was this going to bring me the peace I was looking for finally? Only time would tell. Well, I ended 2015 still single and still looking for some closure. I couldn't figure out what it would take to find that missing piece, but I wasn't giving up on it. In October of 2015, I participated in my first AIDS Walk, and the organization I was walking for asked me to do an interview for a well-known TV Network to help bring awareness to the event. I had previously volunteered to share my story with hopes of finally filling in the missing piece. Maybe the missing piece was **advocacy**[22]? I was so tired of people shaming me or trying to keep me behind closed doors because of my status.

My resolution to that problem was to tell whoever would listen that I had HIV, and then they couldn't say they didn't know. I felt AMAZING after sharing my story and finally getting positive feedback that I wanted to keep going. On December 21st of that year, I wrote a poem on my social media and disclosed my HIV status to the world. It was exhilarating. The post had over four hundred likes and over forty shares. None of the comments were negative like I expected them to be. So, going into 2016, I decided I would host an HIV/AIDS Awareness Gala. I was nervous about doing it but excited at the same time. I was still working on accepting that the person who exposed me to HIV was born with it.

I was still working on accepting that the love I once loved was becoming the love I once knew, and I was still accepting the fact that I was now raising two children all by

---

[22] public support for or recommendation of a particular cause or policy. Oxford Languages

myself. The Gala was the perfect distraction. However, I did not have a date for my own event! There was no way I could show alone, especially as the host of the party. I had ONE LAST fiasco with Alex, and that was our end-all, be-all. I was invited to celebrate New Year's Eve at a hotel with one of his cousins. I knew he would be there, so I made sure I was dressed to a "T." hair done and make up done. That night did NOT go well. It was just awkward being there and feeling like people were whispering about us.

I wanted to address the "elephant in the room," so we ended up talking in the hallway. Well, I talked. I had been drinking and was all in my feelings about everything, and I just lost it. I just ended up expressing how angry I was, how much I hated that I was so in love with him and how all I wanted was for him to be there. In reality, though, he didn't owe me that. He didn't owe me anything. But since I used him as a scapegoat for all these years, I felt very strongly that he owed me SOMETHING. I was wrong. And that would be the last conversation he and I would ever have. I got a friend request in early 2016 from someone I met after leaving Darius for the first time in Atlanta.

His name was Bryce. I accepted his request, and he immediately messages me and asks how I had been. I responded, although I was hesitant to entertain the conversation considering the luck I was having with guys. We started conversing and then all of a sudden, we were talking every day two to three times a day. It was natural, and it was chemistry. It was different this time around. He was living in Louisiana at the time, and I asked him if he wanted to come up to Chicago to be my date for my Gala. He was ecstatic. He couldn't wait to be a part of what I was trying to do. He caught a roundtrip flight, and he came ready to help in whatever way he could.

He was dressed very nicely, and he was very, very polite. Everyone loved him. We had talked so much, and I was so comfortable with him that I didn't want him to leave when it was time for him to go. Yes, I was going through many things, but I felt like I needed him there. I wanted him there, and he wanted to be there. So, guess what? He stayed. It was a huge adjustment for him because I had a three and a five-year-old. He hadn't ever been in a stepparent role. We had many a nights of arguing over things that seemed to be common sense to me, but because he hadn't raised kids, it didn't come naturally for him. I can admit I had high expectations for someone who just uprooted their whole life and moved to Illinois on a whim.

I do think that was a big part of our eventual downfall. We did a lot together and were always down for anything that had to do with me advocating or speaking. He would even speak at some events with me and allow others to ask him questions about what it was like to be with someone who had HIV when he didn't have it. I know I moved fast with him as well. I talked myself into believing that he was marriage material. Who else was going to accept me this way? With two kids with two different dads? Who else was going to come along on my speaking engagements and participate?

No one. I was convinced that this was it. We had a lot of ups and downs. Again, I was still dealing with a lot of demons, and I wasn't ready to admit that I was still grieving in so many different areas of my life. I just wanted to move on. I found consolation in moving forward in my relationship and advocating…Or so I thought. I had assured myself that I would marry him and that I wanted another child with my HUSBAND. I think me still looking for love and closure impacted that decision. At the end of 2016, I had miscarried. After finding out I was pregnant that time, we were excited. So, when we lost it, we tried again for another one. This time, I carried the baby to 36 weeks and had him on my Dad's birthday. Bryce and I were not married when I got pregnant the second time.

However, we wanted to be married before we had him. We thought we would be doing better than what we had done in the past by being married. We got married on August 26th, and my third child was born on September 12th of 2017. I made lots and lots of irrational decisions while seeking solaces in different things and different people. I really wish I had taken the time to talk to more people about what I was going through and how I felt. My marriage failed. I was still the angry woman I was when I was with Isaiah. I was still scared and defensive all the time, and I was absolutely overprotective of my kids.

Bryce wanted to lead and make important decisions in the relationship, but I wasn't ready to give up control. Knowing that I wasn't prepared to pass the baton to him, I shouldn't have gotten into that relationship, and I shouldn't have gotten married. I took vows that I realized I couldn't live up to, and quite honestly, he had a hard time living up to them as well. He felt like I wasn't playing my role as a wife, and I felt like he wasn't playing his part either. One thing you shouldn't expect when you get married is for the relationship to change. If it wasn't that way before, don't expect it to be that way after. Of course, growth happens. That's natural.

You will naturally grow with your partner and continually learn from each other, but there are certain things that you shouldn't expect a marriage to change. The night before he even proposed to me, we got into a huge argument, and I kicked him out and made him sleep in his car. It was twelve degrees outside. I couldn't believe he still wanted to marry me! I felt like I had so much power and control because it was my house, my car, my everything. But there's a meme I found that says, *"If money and material things make you believe you are better than others, you are the poorest person on Earth."* It was wrong and completely unfair for me to kick him out, knowing he had nowhere to go. I was just a woman scorned, and I was just numb to feelings.

I could turn my feelings on and off like a light switch and not think twice about it. I ended up taking on a new role within the company I started working for after I graduated.

Bryce and I wanted a change of scenery, and we wanted OUT of the cold. So, we moved to his hometown in Louisiana. I liked it there, but we didn't do well. Within thirty days of being there, we were arguing way too much. I was second-guessing moving there and being away from my family with three kids. It was hard for him to find work, and I struggled to cover all the expenses on my own. It was a mess, and we were not equipped to take on that kind of stress.

I admit I was a runner. It was easier for me to let it go than to get to the root cause of the problem and fix it. Bryce will tell you to this day that I was looking for an out from that marriage, and maybe he was right? I didn't know what I wanted when I got married. I just thought I was doing what was right. In early 2016, right before my first Gala, I was diagnosed with anxiety and depression. I was severely depressed. I was having a hard time accepting that this was my life. I never got an apology from Darius, and I used Alex as a Scapegoat. I blamed him for everything. I wrote several times in my journals over the years that if we would've just worked it out, I would've never moved to Georgia, and I would've never contracted HIV.

That was such a huge burden for him to carry, and it was one hundred percent not his fault that I was in the position I was in. But I know I pushed those feelings onto him. There was a lot of emotional and verbal abuse in my marriage. It wasn't healthy for either one of us to continue in the marriage. I moved to Texas, and he moved away as well, and we both just wanted to start over. Again, we are closer today than we ever were as a married couple. Accountability was not my area of expertise, and I was blaming everyone but myself for getting HIV and suffering from major depression, anxiety, and PTSD.

I needed to take responsibility for my actions, but I was just too angry to do that. I blamed Darius more than anything and anybody. Yes, I should have been more responsible, but he had an obligation also as a decent human being. Yes, we should have gotten tested before engaging in unprotected sex (this is the accountability part lol) but I thought I learned him enough to trust what he told me. ***The truth is, you can't put ANYTHING past ANYBODY, and you should always know your status and the status of your partner!***

I mean, how do you do what he did and not feel bad about it or even apologize? Here I was once again searching high and low for a consolation that I would never find. In reality, I needed to stop seeking solace in other people and start seeking solace in myself. I needed to seek understanding and try to figure out how I would walk in this new purpose that God was showing me. It started to become clear as day that I was here to share my story with the world and help someone that may be going through what I had gone through over the years.

At the end of the day, all I needed was ME. A put-together me, not a broken me. A PROUD me, not a miserable me. I had to love myself before I could ever love someone else. This realization was so refreshing, and it was only a matter of time before I would feel myself finally starting to reach the top.

'It's funny how you may never know the true effect you may have on somebody else watching your life. In your eyes they may see dreams and hopes and aspirations that might help them want to carry on fighting their fight..."

(Keyshia Cole, Sometimes, Calling All Hearts)

∽ **Believing In Me** ∽

As I said in the beginning, the end of my relationship with my "college sweetheart" was the beginning of my worst nightmare. I went looking for love in all the wrong places and hit many bumps in the road on my journey. Here we are in 2021, and I can officially say I am walking in my purpose. I can officially say that the trials and tribulations that got me here were well worth the heartache and the pain. It took a lot of wrongs for me to get it right. I lost a lot along the way, and I am still learning to cope with many different aspects of my life. I fell in love in 2007, and fourteen years later, I can finally say that I have found my solace, and it wasn't in someone but was in someTHING. It's right here in this book. It's right here within myself. To be good for someone else, you must be good for yourself first. No one wants damaged goods!

Therapy was the best thing I could have done for myself. Until recently, I feel it was frowned upon, and people called you crazy for having mental health issues and needing to talk about it. My diagnosis of Anxiety, PTSD, and Depression answered many questions for me and helped me better learn how to navigate certain challenges. Yes, I take medication for it. Yes, I take medication to control my HIV. And that is OK with me. I used to be embarrassed to carry around pills. I never wanted people to know what I was really going through because I didn't want anyone to judge me. But now, who cares, and who are you to judge? Don't be damaged goods. ***Take time to take care of yourself and embrace self-love and self-care.***

Loving someone so deeply that essentially would never love me the same broke me down. However, it allowed me to build myself back up with all those broken pieces. I had to move around. I had to get a change of scenery. I had to go through mentally, physically, and emotionally abusive relationships to understand what I was worth and what I deserved. That was MY story. That is not EVERYONE'S story and I am by no means condoning the abuse. I had to experience those to understand the role I played in my own healing process. If you don't acknowledge that there is pain and that you are hurting, you will have a tough time seeing yourself through. For you to fix it, you first have to admit that it's broken. This was not a walk in the park for me.

This book was by no means easy to write. It opened wounds that I healed from and moved on from. It brought back very traumatizing experiences that I STILL seek therapy for today. It's not something that happens, and you just get over it…and it's OK NOT to be OK! HIV doesn't discriminate; it's not going to skip someone because they have a million dollars, and it's not going to skip someone because they only have a dollar. If you engage in the activities that could cause you to contract the virus, you are just as vulnerable as anyone else.

I took my lemons, and I made lemonade. I am aware that not everyone can do that. I don't feel like I will ever get justice for what was done to me, but I've accepted that. I channeled that energy and put it into doing positive things like bringing awareness to my story by writing this book. I find great joy in spending time with my children and traveling. *I got another chance to get it right, and if you are still here and reading this, then you have another chance too.* I was a prisoner of my own mind for a very long time. I was suffering in silence with mental health disorders and my chronic illness.

I was uneducated in thinking HIV is AIDS, that I didn't have much longer to live. Education is key, and it will take you far if you let it. A lot of people ask me things like, *"How did I make it? How do I get through my days?"* The truth is, I know this isn't my end all, be all. I know that even with HIV, I can still be great. I got my bachelor's degree at twenty-seven. I have three children in which none of them contracted HIV. I knew the importance of adherence to my medication, not just for the sake of not passing the virus to my kids and partner, but also for trying to keep my viral load undetectable.

That's how I make it through my days. I went back for my degree with an eighteen-month-old, got pregnant in the first semester, and I STILL PUSHED THROUGH. It's essential to not set limitations on yourself. You have to have those positive affirmations. No one can believe in you more than you believe in yourself. I am a true survivor of HIV. I am

SURVIVING HIV still, and I am making sure I pave the way for those who think they can't make it through one more day. You must find an outlet and use it to your advantage! For instance, of all the months out of the year, December is HIV Awareness month. December is also Christmas! December is also the month that I found out I had HIV.

So, while it's an exciting time for most, it's a constant reminder of what we have been through for some of us. Things that help me get through the holidays is traveling. It helps to keep my mind and body busy. It also makes me feel revived when I'm celebrating with other people. I also enjoy doing crafts with my kids and writing poetry. I started hosting HIV/AIDS Awareness events to deal with my living with HIV as well. I wanted to share my story to let people know that I contracted HIV from someone that "loved" me. I wasn't promiscuous, and having a high GPA, a good-paying job, and being a good Samaritan didn't stop me from getting it.

The medication is expensive! You don't want to put that price tag on your life! I've learned how to forgive, but I'll never forget. I've learned to embrace this circumstance and make one hell of a journey out of it, and you should too! I don't care what people think about me because I have HIV. I made it my duty to empower those going through my struggle. No one deserves to be mistreated or discriminated against based on their HIV status. I've been given a beautiful platform to share my story. I have been afforded so many opportunities that will help change the way people look at HIV.

Contracting HIV was the most humbling experience I have ever had in my life. I grew up privileged. I got good grades in school. I was kind to people, and I was faithful. And if ANY of those things mattered when I contracted HIV, then maybe I wouldn't have it. But the fact of that matter is that NONE OF THAT MATTERS WHEN IT COMES TO HIV. Contracting HIV has taught me patience; it has shown me ignorance; it has taught me to educate, advocate, and be understanding. It took the normalcy out of my life and, in the same breath, made it OK to be a little different.

It has inspired me to become an Author, and in writing this book, I realized so much about people. I've loved, and I've lost along the way, but the sacrifice has been worth it. My biggest goal that I hope to achieve over the years is to erase the stigma and the shame associated with HIV/AIDS. It may not be your life, but it's mine and millions of other people's. I want my book to be carried in hospitals and HIV clinics all around the world! And If I can save just one life by telling my story, I will tell it over and over and over again. The most rewarding part of this journey is getting those emails, those @'s on social media of people tagging you with positive things they found about you or to simply let you know that they are inspired. Its fulfilling to know they made it another day because of your story.

You never know who your story can help, but I encourage you always to speak up. Another thing is it's essential to have a positive support system and positive role models. Keep people around you who encourage you and challenge you to go to great lengths. I had the very best friends that helped me through a lot of my situations. Some of them I knew before I had HIV, and some I met along the way. But they always told me the truth whether I wanted to hear it or not. They always gave me good advice (whether I took it or not was on me.) And when I bumped my head, they never said, *"I told you so..."* They supported me, comforted me when I needed it, and they still are a very active and necessary part of my life.

I remember nights I would fall asleep after a long day at work and school, and Tiffany would come over and close my blinds and turn all my lights off. She had a key to my house. I have another friend Shae that I would drop my babies off to when I got overwhelmed and couldn't get them to stop crying. She already had two children before I had my second one, and I just felt like she knew everything. I would call her for everything from constipation to ear infections. She was and still is the most kind and patient person I have ever met. We were all college students with families with the same end goal, and we helped each other whenever and wherever we could. We helped pick up and drop off for daycare; we had ladies' night and couple's nights (drinking some nights followed by games and movies another.)

I would've never made it without my small circle of people. **Do not underestimate the need for positive friendships/relationships.** Friendships that grow with you and not hinder you. I used to feel like it was hard and inconvenient having friends that didn't have kids! It was like anxiety for me when I had children. I used to think, *"she's not going to want to come over and hang out, listening to crying babies or me say 'stop that' or 'put that down' all evening..."* But I was so wrong! **DON'T THINK LIKE THAT! PEOPLE LOVE YOU! PEOPLE LOVE YOUR KIDS!** Even if they don't have any! My best friend Ashley since the sixth grade doesn't have children yet, and she loves me and everything that comes with me. Real friends understand your baggage, embrace it, and help you lighten the load!

I found this meme on social media that said, *"If you don't learn the difference between someone who is against you and someone who challenges you, you'll be pushing away nourishment for your soul to embrace those who will starve it..."* I couldn't agree more. I most certainly had people that were draining me, and I didn't even realize it. I no longer associate with those people! Don't let anyone starve your soul, and you make sure you aren't starving theirs! Another positive change I made was a choice to be **celibate**[23]. This has been one of the more difficult decisions I have made. The truth is, I have been giving bits and pieces of myself for SO many years. I decided I wanted to keep me FOR ME

---

[23] *Not engaging in or characterized by sexual intercourse.* merriam-webster.com

until I can give my WHOLE self to someone, physically and emotionally.

One last thing that helped me along the way and still helps me today is music. Music was a huge part of my journey through grief and HIV. *Albums like Passion, Pain, and Pleasure by Trey Songz, Jazmine Sullivan's "Love Me Back" or Keyshia Cole's "Calling All Hearts"* all spoke to me in different ways. Sometimes, I would play them and write in my journal and be able to tune out everyone and everything. The album that impacted me the most was *Monica's "Still Standing" album,* which came out not too long after I tested positive. When I say I can barely listen to that album to this day and not cry, I am not exaggerating. I had to continually remind myself that I was STILL STANDING and show the world that there was a reason I was STILL STANDING.

Her music before and after that album was always so relatable to me. This album, in particular, came when I didn't know which way my life was going or if I would make it to the end of 2010. I listened to *"Still Standing"* repeatedly...She says, *"I been through the storm, had dirt on my name, I'm still holding on, Champion of the game..."* I was still holding on. After everything I had been through, I was still standing. Her, *"Believing in me"* song was a tear-jerker and the last song on her album. I would guess that was intentional. It was like the firework finale on the Fourth of July. For me, the part where she says, *"I hope you can forgive me. I'm not gonna be the way that I used to be.*

Starting over can be so scary, but I'm gonna believe. Promise, I'm not gonna let me down, and my transformation's starting right now..." was her declaration.

Just as much as it was a declaration for her, it was a declaration for me too. Sometimes, we just have to remind ourselves that starting over isn't always easy but definitely worth it. We have to have faith that there is something greater waiting for us. It does get greater later. **Dr. Martin Luther King Jr. said it best,** *"Faith is taking the first step even if you don't see the whole staircase."*

So, take the first step. Your mind, body, and soul will thank you for it.

✑ **About The Author** ✑

Jessica Glaspie is a well-known HIV Advocate with features running in some of the most widely circulated magazines internationally and domestically.

She calls the Dallas-Fort Worth area home for now but travels back to the Chicagoland area often to visit family and friends. She loves to travel with her family and eat! Her favorite food is none other than a good Ol' Chicago-style stuffed pizza.

Visit her website: www.lifeloveandhiv.com to book speaking engagements and follow her blog as she talks about everyday things and emotions while journeying through life with HIV.

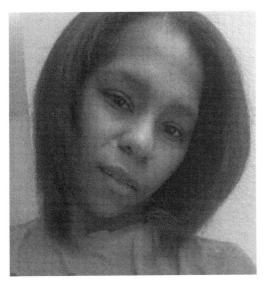

IG: Shewearsitwelltoo
FB: Life, Love and HIV (Personal Blog)
Youtube: Life, Love, and HIV
Twitter: JGlaspie1

Follow the Life, Love, and HIV playlist on Spotify!

#TeamJessica #SheWearsItWell #LifeLoveAndHIV

Made in the USA
Columbia, SC
21 March 2021